PAIN IS NOT YOUR HOME

Your Roadmap to Freedom and Unshakable Worth

AROHA RIPLEY

Pain is Not Your Home: Your roadmap to unshakable worth
Aroha Ripley

First published in Australia © 2026 Aroha Ripley
All rights reserved.

arohaRipley.com

ISBN (Print):   978-0-6458793-3-9
ISBN (eBook): 978-0-6458793-4-6

Cover design: Aroha Ripley
Interior typeset & design: Beckon Creative, Aroha Ripley
Printed in Australia

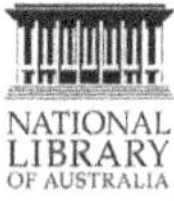

A catalogue record for this book is available from the National Library of Australia

Disclaimer Notice: This book is based on personal experience and spiritual reflection and is not intended to be a substitute for professional medical, psychological, or psychiatric advice, diagnosis, or treatment.

Please consult a qualified professional for all health-related concerns. If you are in crisis, contact your local emergency services immediately.

KO WAI AU — Who am I?

Ko Taranaki te maunga
Ko Kapuni te awa
Ko Te Aroha o Tītokowaru te marae
Ko Ngāruahine te iwi
Ko Aroha Ripley ahau

Tēnā koutou katoa.

Kia ora,
My name is Aroha.

I stand grounded in my whakapapa
in the strength, the story,
and the truth of where I come from.

I carry the legacy of those before me.
I carry the lessons that shaped me.

I have walked through pain.
I have sat in darkness.
I have carried what was never mine to carry.

I know what it is to survive
and I chose not to stay there.

I am still standing.

This is where I come from.
This is what I stand on.

Pain is not my home.

CONTENTS

Dedication

For those who have carried pain they never asked for. For the ones who learned how to smile while breaking inside.
For those who felt unseen, unheard, or not enough.

And for the ones who, even in the darkness, held a small hope that life could be different.

This book is for you.

Pain is not your home.
Healing is.

Acknowledgments

This book is a testimony to what can be rebuilt when you refuse to give up. It exists because of the hands and the heart of the One who never let me go, and the unconditional love of my whānau and friends.

To Jesus My Lord and Saviour:

Thank You for refusing to let me stay in the dark. Thank You for taking the pieces that broke me and turning them into the foundation of my purpose. This book is proof that You are near the brokenhearted, and I owe every ounce of my healing and strength to Your unfailing love and grace.

To My Beloved Whānau:

To my husband, my anchor and my best friend, thank you for standing with me, for your love, patience, and unwavering support on the days I struggled the most. Your presence has carried me farther than words can ever express.

To my children, daughters-in-law, and mokopuna (grandchildren), you are my heart and my why. Every step I take, every boundary I set, and every risk I embrace is for you. May this book remind you that no matter the pain you face, courage, love, and purpose are always possible. Never stop chasing your dreams.

FOREWORD

A Personal Message from Aroha

If you are holding this book in a moment of deep pain, I want you to pause for a second and breathe. You don't need to have the right words. You don't need to know what comes next. You only need to know this: **you are not alone, and this book was written with you in mind.**

When pain stays for a long time, it can start to feel familiar. It can feel like something you have to live with, something you have to carry, something you have to call home. But pain was never meant to be where you stay. **Pain is not your home.**

You may be tired in ways that are hard to explain.
You may feel lost, numb, or overwhelmed.
You may be wondering if life will ever feel lighter again.

Nothing is wrong with you for feeling this way.

This book is not here to pressure you to heal quickly or to pretend everything is okay. It is here to walk beside you, gently and honestly, as you begin to remember who you are underneath the hurt.

These pages were written for the moments when hope feels far away. For the nights when the weight feels too heavy. For the quiet questions you may be afraid to ask. They are here to remind you that even if pain has been part of your story, it does not get to decide your future.

You don't have to leave your pain all at once. You don't have to be strong today. You only have to take one small step, and sometimes that step is simply turning the page.

Let this book be a resting place, not a demand. A reminder, not a judgment. A gentle truth whispered back to you again and again: **you were never meant to live here. There is a way forward. And you are worthy of finding it.**

Much love,

Aroha Ripley xx

INTRODUCTION

The Journey Begins

My friend, take a deep breath. You made it here, and that means a part of you still believes there's more to life than pain. Stop apologising for your pain, stop hiding your tears, and open these pages. Let this book meet you exactly where you are.

Trauma is real, and healing is messy. I'm not here to tell you to "just get over it." I know the depth of that pain because I've walked this road barefoot. I won't lie to you or offer quick fixes. Instead, I offer you this truth: **Pain is a teacher, not a tenant.** It may have barged in through heartbreak, loss, or fear, but it doesn't have to condemn you. I am here, not above you, but **beside you,** to hold space for the work ahead, in a space of truth, compassion, and non-judgment.

This book is not about ignoring the broken pieces; it's about learning how to transform them. It is your roadmap, a clear, uncompromising pathway out of pain and into **freedom.**

Over the coming pages, you will find tools, reflection prompts, and real steps to shift your story. When the dust clears, you'll declare with unshakable certainty: **"Pain is not my home. Freedom is."** To get there, you'll learn how to:

- Confront what hurts without being consumed by it.

- Break free from old stories that say you're not enough.

- Understand how fear and doubt keep showing up.

- Rebuild your confidence from the inside out.

Be gentle with yourself. Healing isn't a race; it's a journey of **progress, not perfection.** I want you to read slowly, cry if you need to, and rest when it feels heavy. Because pain might have knocked at your door, but it doesn't get to own the house. **You do.**
It's time to release, reclaim, rebuild, and return home to the truest version of you. Welcome home, my beautiful friend. Let's begin.

DISCLAIMER

Disclaimer & Notice

This book is a labor of love and a reflection of my own journey and coaching experience. While I am a business and transformation coach dedicated to helping others find their way out of the dark, I am not a licensed psychologist, psychiatrist, counselor, or medical professional. The contents of this book are for **educational, spiritual, and informational purposes only.**

The "way home" looks different for everyone. The insights and strategies shared here are not intended to diagnose, treat, or cure any mental health condition or clinical disorder. This book is meant to be a companion to, not a replacement for, professional medical or psychological care.

If you are in a crisis, struggling with deep-seated clinical trauma, or feeling that your life is in danger, please do not go it alone. Reach out to a licensed professional, a mental health clinic, or a crisis hotline immediately. There is no shame in needing a higher level of care; in fact, seeking it is one of the most powerful steps you can take toward your own return.

By reading this book, you acknowledge that you are responsible for your own choices and well-being. My hand is reaching out to help you stand, but the path you walk is yours.

For crisis support numbers, please see the end of this book.

PART ONE

Release

Evicting the Past
and Finding the Courage to Stop Running

CHAPTER 1

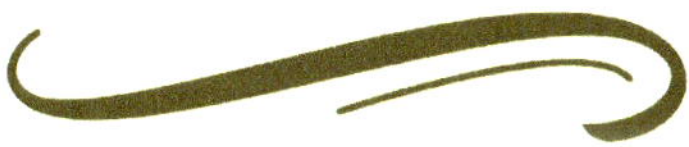

WELCOME HOME: CHOOSING TO BEGIN

Pain is a teacher, not a tenant.

THE INVITATION:
I See You Standing at the Door

There comes a moment when you finally realize you can't keep carrying what broke you.

Maybe it crept in quietly, through tears no one ever saw. Maybe it hit all at once, when the weight of it all became unbearable.
Either way, you're here. And that matters.

Your heart knows the truth, even if your mind is still trying to catch up. It's been whispering all along: you were made for more.

This isn't about pretending the pain never happened. It happened. And it hurts. And it left its mark.

AROHA RIPLEY

But here's the thing: the pain doesn't get to stay.
It doesn't get to define you.
It doesn't get to decide your story.

You are not just what broke you.
You are not the fear, the shame, the exhaustion,
the rejection.

You are more.
So much more than what tried to take you down.

And right here, right now, this is where your story
starts again.

MY STORY:
I've Walked This Road Barefoot

If you've never heard my story before, let me give you a little insight into who I am, and why I wrote *Pain Is Not Your Home.*

I didn't write this book from a place of comfort or theory. I wrote it from lived experience. From nights where the pain felt louder than my hope. From seasons where survival was the goal, not purpose. From a life shaped by wounds I never chose, but carried for far too long.

I know pain, not as a concept, but as something that lived in my body, my thoughts, my spirit. I know what it's like to feel unseen, unwanted, and exhausted from being "strong." I know what it's like to question God, to feel distant from Him, to wonder if He sees you or hears you at all. I know what it's like to sit with shame, fear, and silence and wonder if this is just how life is meant to be.

For a long time, pain felt like home to me. Familiar. Normal. Expected.
But deep down, something in me knew, this couldn't be it.

No one invites pain into their life.

It doesn't ask permission.
It doesn't wait for you to be ready.
It doesn't explain itself.

It arrives without warning, quietly at first, then all at once, often when you are most vulnerable, when your guard is down, when you are still learning who you are. One moment you're living, and the next you're carrying something you never agreed to hold.

When I look back now, I can see that my pain wasn't one moment or one event. It came in layers. One wound stacked on top of another. Loss after loss. Rejection. Hardship. Moments that slowly stripped away my sense of safety, my identity, and my belief that I mattered. At the time, I didn't have the language for what was happening inside me. I just knew something was breaking, quietly and deeply.

Some of my deepest wounds began in childhood, through words spoken by the one person who was meant to nurture, protect, and love me, my mother.

"You will never become anything."
"You are useless."
"No one will want you."

Those words didn't just hurt in the moment. They stayed. They settled into my heart and made themselves at home. They became the lens through which I saw myself. They became the voice in my head, the one that followed me into every room, every relationship, every dream.

When your own mother tells you she didn't want you because you were a girl, it leaves a mark that doesn't fade with time. It shapes how you love, how you trust, how you show up in the world. It teaches you, without saying it out loud, that love is conditional, and that you are somehow lacking.

I didn't choose this pain.
I was a child.

What I carried was never my fault, but it was placed on me through words, through silence, through rejection, emotional abuse, and sexual abuse, experiences no child should ever have to survive, let alone carry into adulthood. Yet I did. Quietly. Alone. Doing the best I could with what I had.

Insecurity became my constant companion. It followed me like a shadow, always there, always whispering that I wasn't enough. And when pain is ignored for too long, it doesn't disappear, it finds louder ways to be felt.

For me, it showed up as depression, anxiety, fear, explosions of anger and a bone-deep exhaustion that rest couldn't fix.
A heaviness in my chest I couldn't explain.
A constant searching, for relief, for answers, for something to numb the ache, the pain and the voices in my head.

I felt disconnected from myself, from others, and from God.

I was raised knowing about who God and Jesus are, but what I experienced behind closed doors didn't reflect His love. That contradiction created distance. Confusion. Anger. I found myself asking questions I didn't know how to say out loud: *How could You let this happen to me? What did I do wrong? What did I do to deserve this pain from the people who were meant to love me? Where are You, Jesus?*

I knew He was real, but I was hurting so deeply that even praying felt impossible.

On the outside, I was functioning. I was showing up, going with the flow, I was surviving, hiding behind my smile just to please everyone else.
But on the inside, I wasn't free, I was in turmoil.

The weight of guilt, shame, and the relentless voices in my mind became unbearable. There were moments I truly believed the world would be better without me. Survival became my only goal, getting through the next hour, let alone the next day. I felt invisible. Like my voice didn't matter. Like my pain didn't count. I believed the lies that taunted me daily, that I was worth nothing, no one loved me or cared about me.

But even in my darkest moments, there was a quiet voice that wouldn't leave me alone.
Soft. Steady. Persistent.

You are worthy.
You were created for a purpose.
You are loved.
Don't give up on yourself.

And that's when I knew something had to change.
I couldn't keep carrying what broke me and still call it strength.
I couldn't keep surviving and pretend it was living.

So I stopped running.

I stopped pretending I was okay when I wasn't.
I stopped lying to myself.
I stopped letting pain live in places it was never meant to stay.

I stopped searching for validation from my mother and from others, even when my sense of worth lay in pieces at my feet. I reached a place of desperation, not only for answers, but for peace. Real peace. The kind that doesn't depend on approval, performance, or pretending. The kind only God can give.

And it was there, not when everything was fixed, not when I felt strong or faithful, that God met me.

Not with judgement.
Not with conditions.
But with His unconditional love.

He met me in my tears.
In the silence.
In the mess I didn't know how to clean up.

Slowly, gently, I began to realize I wasn't abandoned. That even in my confusion, my questioning, my brokenness, I was still held. My wairua, my spirit, knew before my mind could catch up:

I am not alone.

Pain is part of life.
No one escapes it. Not in the body. Not in the mind. Not in the heart.

You can ignore it for a while.
Push it down.
Tell yourself you're fine.

But pain doesn't disappear just because you refuse
to look at it. It waits.
And when it's been ignored for too long, it finds a way
to be felt.

I finally realized that while pain is a part of life, it
doesn't get to rule my life. It might knock on my door,
but it doesn't get to move in and stay. Finding that
truth was the awakening I didn't know I needed.

I'm here with you now not because I figured
everything out,
but because I've sat in the mess.

I've carried pain longer than I should have.
And I made a choice: not to stay there.

I chose life.
Even when it scared me.
Even when it felt unfamiliar.
Even when I didn't trust myself yet.

I chose to say yes to the opportunities placed in front of me,
the small ones and the life-changing ones.
The ones that stretched me.
The ones that asked me to believe there could be more.

I stopped letting pain define me.
I stopped letting it decide what I deserved.

I stopped surrounding myself with toxic people and words.

I realized that I wasn't just here to occupy space or to endure pain. I had to find my **"Why."** I had to understand the reason I was still breathing after everything I'd been through. This wasn't just a change of pace; it was the start of a journey to find my purpose, the one that had been waiting for me to stop running long enough to catch it.

This book was born out of that knowledge. Out of the moment I realized that pain may be part of my story, but it was never meant to be my permanent address. Pain is a place you pass through, not where you belong. That surviving wasn't the same as living. And that healing, real healing, begins when you stop running from the truth and start facing it with honesty, courage, and faith.

I'm not here as someone who has it all together. I'm here as someone who has been broken, questioned everything, wrestled with God, and still chose life. Someone who learned, step by step, that pain can teach you, but it doesn't get to stay.

Pain Is Not Your Home exists because I believe with everything in me that if healing was possible for me, it is possible for you too. And if you're reading this right now, it's not by accident.

THE TRUTH:
Pain is a Teacher, Not a Tenant

When you feel unseen, unheard, or like your worth slipped through the cracks, it's easy to believe the lie that you have to stay small or stay silent. You may have tried everything to stop the ache: working harder, staying busy, pretending you're okay, or just pushing through. But the emptiness doesn't fade.

And I need you to hear this truth: Pain is a teacher, not a tenant.

It is not here to condemn you; it is here to reveal what still needs healing. It forces us to stop running and finally see the quiet strength underneath all the exhaustion we've been faking. The fact that you picked up this book is proof that something in you refuses to give up.

THE REALITY CHECK:
Your Brain is Just Trying to Keep You Safe

Your brain remembers pain because it's trying to protect you. It's wired to keep you safe, not necessarily happy. That's why one word, smell, or place can bring old feelings rushing back, even years later. Your brain isn't punishing you, it just doesn't realize the danger has passed.

Here's the hope: Your brain can learn new patterns. When you face pain gently, one piece at a time, you teach it: **"I can feel this and still be okay."**

Each time you choose honesty over fear, your mind learns safety again. Healing isn't just emotional, it's physical too.

THE DRILL:
Finding Your Breath in the Storm (Calm Practice)

When painful thoughts or emotions start to rise, your nervous system can panic and think you're in danger even when you're not. This practice will help calm your body and remind your brain that you are safe right now.

1. **Pause and Notice.** Stop for a moment. Notice your breath, your heartbeat, your feet on the ground. Just become aware of where you are right now.

2. **Remind Yourself You're Safe.** Gently tell yourself: **"I'm safe in this moment."** You don't have to feel completely calm yet, this is just a reminder to your brain that the danger has passed.

3. **Breathe with Intention.** Take a slow breath in through your nose, hold for two seconds, and breathe out through your mouth. Repeat three times. Slow breathing tells your nervous system it's okay to relax.

4. **Name What You Feel.** Say quietly to yourself: "This is sadness." "This is fear." "This is grief." Naming the feeling helps your brain understand it's just an emotion, not a threat.

5. **Focus on What Is Real and Steady.** Find something around you that feels solid and calming, the chair beneath you, the floor under your feet, or the sound of your breathing. Let your focus stay there for a few moments.

6. **Bring Kindness into the Moment.** Think of one small thing that feels comforting, a person, a pet, a memory, or a simple truth like **"I've made it through hard things before."** Let that thought soften your body and heart.

Every time you do this, you're teaching your brain a new truth: **"I can feel pain and still be safe."** Over time, your mind learns peace as a habit, one calm breath, one kind thought at a time.

THE HARD QUESTIONS:
What Are You Tired of Carrying?

It's time to get real. No more skimming the surface. No more pretending. Let's shine a light on the weight you've been dragging, sometimes without even realizing it.

Ask yourself:

1. What lies am I still believing about myself that aren't true?

2. What shame have I been carrying that isn't mine to own?

3. What anger, hurt, or betrayal have I locked away instead of facing?

4. Who or what have I been trying to fix, control, or forgive, when really it's their responsibility, not mine?

5. What pain am I holding onto because I'm scared to let it go?

6. How has pretending I'm "okay" cost me my voice, my freedom, my joy?

7. What would it take to release the weight that has been keeping me small, stuck, or silent?

Take a deep breath. Sit with each one. You don't have to answer them all at once. Some will bring tears. Some will bring anger. Some will bring relief. That's okay.

The questions aren't meant to punish you, they're meant to wake you up. To wake you up to the life you were made for. To the strength, courage, and freedom that's already inside you, waiting to be claimed.
Because the moment you face even one of these truths... that's the moment you take back your power.

THE COMMITMENT:
I Am Showing Up for Me

Today, I am making a choice to stop running. I've spent too much time fleeing from my past and hiding from my potential, but the race ends here. I am finally showing up for myself, and for today, that is enough.

I am learning to breathe again. Slowly. Deeply. Freely. I am letting go of the pressure to be perfect and the need to have every answer. I finally accept the truth: Pain is a teacher, not a tenant. My hurt may have taught me how to survive, but it is not my home, and it no longer has permission to live in my future. Even in the middle of my doubt and fear, I am choosing to heal.

Signed, ____

(No more excuses. No more waiting. This is who I am now.)

THE FINAL CHARGE:
You've Got the Power to Begin Again

You are not your past. You are not the pain. You are the person who survived it and that's where your power begins.

So as you open your heart to this journey, let go of the idea that you need to have it all together. You don't. All you need is a willingness to begin again.

This is your invitation to rise, to reclaim your worth, rediscover your voice, and remember that God has not finished your story.

Pain is not my home. Freedom is.

THE SEAL:
A Prayer for Your New Beginning

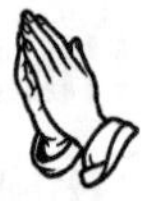

Dear Heavenly Father,

I may not know you fully but I come to You with all the pieces of me that have been broken, scattered, and heavy. I don't have it all together. I am tired, I am raw, I am hurting. But I need You.

Thank You for holding me even when I felt invisible, for meeting me in my tears, and for showing me that I am not alone. Thank You for turning my pain into purpose, my fear into courage, and my brokenness into a chance to rise again.

Help me to believe that I am enough, that I am loved, and that even in my mess, You are with me. Teach me to release the weight I've been carrying, to trust Your presence, and to walk into the life I was always made for.

In Jesus' Name,
Amen

*"The Lord is close to the brokenhearted
and saves those who are crushed in spirit."*

— *Psalm 34:18* NIV

My Notes

Date: ___________

My Notes

Date: _______________

My Notes

Date: ___________

My Notes

Date: ___________

47

CHAPTER 2

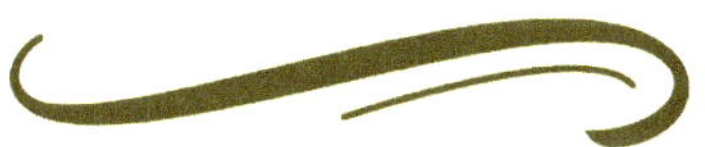

QUIT TRIPPING YOURSELF

Stop self-sabotage. Start living.

THE INVITATION:
Stop Standing in Your Own Way

Let's be honest: sometimes the hardest person to face is the one in the mirror — you.

You talk about healing, you pray for change, but when it's time to take the next step, to accept the love, an act of kindness or generosity or to step into new opportunities, you freeze, you pull back, or you find a reason to walk away. Does that constant reply, "It's not for me, give it to someone else who needs it," sound familiar? You've become an expert at self-sabotage and survival; you know how to keep going when everything hurts, how to smile while you're breaking, and how to hold everyone else together while falling apart yourself. But when it comes to facing you, that's where it gets uncomfortable. You're not broken beyond repair; you've just been living in defense mode for too long. It's time to stop running from the truth and quit tripping over yourself.

MY STORY:
The Queen of Self-Sabotage

I need you to hear me, really hear me. I'm not speaking to you from a pedestal, and I'm not hand-delivering advice from a place of perfection. I am speaking to you from the trenches. I am speaking to you as the former Queen of Self-Sabotage.

For years, I was a master architect. I didn't build a life; I built a fortress. I had the perfect excuses, the right answers, and a smile that functioned like a "Keep Out" sign. I used my warmth as a weapon to keep you at a distance. I would tell myself, "Just smile, Aroha. Keep the mask straight. Because if they see the mess underneath, they're gone."

The Masters of My House

The truth is, I stayed in my world of pain because I was addicted to the certainty of it. Pain was predictable; joy was a threat. I had been mentored by the most brutal masters: **Lies, Hurt, and Fear.** They taught me a logic that felt like safety but tasted like slow poison: *If you reject them first, they can't reject you. If you fail on purpose, you don't have to worry about failing by accident.* I became so guarded that even a kind word felt like an attack. I was so wrapped in the armor of my past that I couldn't feel the warmth of the present. The moment a glimpse of hope appeared, a job opportunity, a real friend, a moment of peace, I didn't embrace it and I didn't trust it. I sabotaged it. I would find a reason to pick a fight, make up excuses, or disappear. I was burning bridges before I even had the courage to put a foot on them. I was the one holding the matches, wondering why I was always stranded.

The Ghost of "Fine"

I lived in a constant state of "Defense Mode." I was the Queen of Disguises and the CEO of "Fake It Till You Make It." If you asked me about my dreams, I wouldn't give you an answer, I would give you tears. Not because I didn't have dreams, but because I was terrified of them.

The voices in my head, the ones that told me I was useless, that I'd never be anything, that I was broken beyond repair, had become my internal compass. I was drowning in a storm of self-limiting beliefs, and I had stayed under for so long that "breathing" felt like a foreign concept.

I wasn't just going through a hard time. I was actively choosing my survival kit over my destiny. I thought my sabotage was keeping me safe, but it was actually keeping me small. It was keeping me alone. It was keeping me in a home that was never meant for me.

The Mirror Moment

I'm sharing this because I know the weight of that crown. I know the exhaustion of pretending. I know what it's like to be your own worst enemy and your own primary obstacle.

I was tripping myself because I was terrified of what would happen if I actually stood up straight. I was choosing the "safety" of my misery over the "unfamiliarity" of my healing.

Does this sound familiar? Are you currently holding the matches to your own future? Are you tripping yourself because you're scared of how far you might actually go if you stopped falling?

You aren't protecting yourself; you're imprisoning yourself. It's time to stop surviving the wreckage and start crossing the bridge. It's time to quit tripping yourself.

THE TRUTH:
Self-Sabotage is a Weed

Self-sabotage is a weed that grows in the dark corners where pain was never healed and truth was never faced. It's the shadow that follows you when you refuse to turn on the light. We tell ourselves we are being careful, but the reality is much harsher: You cannot conquer what you continue to excuse.

For so long, I treated my pain like a permanent resident in my heart. I gave it a key, a room, and a seat at the table. I let it dictate the rules of my house. But I had to learn the hard way that pain was only meant to be a teacher, passing through to give me a lesson in resilience, it was never meant to be my tenant.

The Illusion of Control

Why do we do it? Why do we trip ourselves right when things start to look up? Because self-sabotage feels safer than disappointment. There is a twisted sense of power in being the one to pull the plug. It's the logic of the wounded: It's easier to ruin something yourself than to wait for it to ruin you.

If you fail because you didn't try, you can protect your ego. If you push a good person away, you don't have to worry about them eventually leaving. You think you're in control, but you're actually just a prisoner of your own "what-ifs."

Fear in Disguise

This is the great deception of fear: it dresses itself up as **protection.** It puts on a suit and tie and calls itself "wisdom." It wears a watch and calls itself "bad timing."

- You say, "I'm just being realistic," but you're actually being cynical.

- You say, "I'm waiting for the right moment," but you're actually just paralyzed.

- You say, "I'm protecting my peace," but you're actually just isolating your soul.

Deep down, in the quiet spaces of your mind, you know the truth: Fear is running the show. It has hijacked your intuition and turned it into a weapon against your own progress. You aren't "playing it safe"; you are playing it small.

Evicting the Tenant

To stop tripping yourself, you have to stop lying to yourself. You have to look at those walls you've built and realize they aren't keeping the world out, they are keeping you in. You have to acknowledge that your "survival kit" has become a coffin.

Pain may have been your first language, but it doesn't have to be your last. It's time to stop making excuses for the habits that are holding you hostage. It's time to stop letting a ghost from your past occupy the space meant for your future. The lease is up. It's time to evict the fear and reclaim your home.

THE REALITY CHECK:
Your Brain is Hardwired

We need to have a serious conversation about that armor you're wearing. You know the set, the one made of sarcasm, distance, "low expectations," and hyper-independence. You put it on years ago because the world was cold and people were unpredictable. Back then, that armor saved your life. It was your shield against the arrows of rejection and the fire of betrayal.

But here is the hard reality: The armor you built to protect yourself from old hurt is now the very thing keeping new healing out. You think you're wearing it for protection, but you've actually built a cage. Armor doesn't just stop the bad stuff from getting in; it stops the good stuff from getting out. It keeps you from feeling the warmth of a genuine hug, the sincerity of a compliment, and the light of a new beginning. You are suffocating inside a suit of armor that was meant for one single fight, not for the rest of your life.

Compassion for the Survivor

I want you to hear me clearly: You made those choices back then out of pain, not weakness. Stop beating yourself up for the version of you that did whatever it took to stay alive. You weren't "stupid" for trusting the wrong person, and you weren't "weak" for shrinking yourself to avoid a conflict. You were a survivor. You were doing the best you could with the broken tools you had.

True freedom begins the moment you realize you don't have to keep punishing yourself for who you were when you were just trying to survive. You are not that person anymore, and the war you were fighting is over.

The Familiarity Trap

Here is the biological glitch: Your brain doesn't care if you're happy; it only cares that you're safe. And to your brain, "safe" means "familiar." If you grew up in chaos, peace feels like a threat because it's foreign. If you were raised on criticism, a compliment feels like a trap. Your brain is hardwired to keep you in the environment it recognizes, even if that environment is a prison cell. This is why you sabotage. The moment things get "too good," your internal alarm system goes off. It screams, "This isn't the plan! This isn't what we know!" and you subconsciously reach for the self-destruct button just to get back to the familiar discomfort of the "old you."

Breaking the Wiring

You have to start outsmarting your own survival instincts. You have to tell your brain, "Thank you for trying to protect me, but I am not in danger anymore. I am in growth." It's going to feel uncomfortable. It's going to feel "wrong" to be happy, to be consistent, and to be open. Your brain will tell you that you're "tripping," but the reality is you're finally walking upright.

You aren't a victim of your biology, and you aren't a slave to your past. You are the architect of what happens next. The cage is open, and the only thing keeping you inside is the fear that the sky is too big.

It's time to stop honoring your history at the expense of your destiny.

THE DRILL:

Finding Your Breath in the Storm (The Pause Practice)

You break the pattern every time you show up instead of shut down. Use the **Pause Practice** to interrupt the loop:

1. **Pause and Notice:** When you feel the urge to pull away or create chaos, stop and notice your racing thoughts.

2. **Name the Pattern:** Say gently, "This is my old pattern of self-sabotage," and remind yourself you don't have to react that way anymore.

3. **Breathe and Ground:** Take a slow breath and place your feet firmly on the ground.

4. **Reframe the Need:** Ask, "What do I really need right now? Comfort, clarity, or connection?".

5. **Move Gently:** Take one tiny action that goes against the pattern.

THE HARD QUESTIONS:
What Are You Tired of Carrying?

I need you to get quiet for a moment. No distractions, no "fake it till you make it" energy, just you and the truth. Healing is a selective guest; it won't enter a room where honesty isn't invited. You can't heal what you refuse to look at, and you can't transform what you keep pretending isn't there.

It's time to stop the "polite" internal dialogue. It's time to ask the questions that sting, because the sting is how you know you've hit a nerve that's still alive. If you're tired of tripping over the same stones, you have to be willing to look at your own feet.

Ask yourself these, and don't look away from the answers:

1. **The "Why Wait" Audit:** What is the specific "Master Excuse" I keep on speed-dial to delay my own growth? (Is it "I'm not ready," "It's not the right time," or "I'm just being realistic"?)

2. **The Panic Point:** When life actually starts feeling good, when the water is calm and the sun is out, what part of me panics, and what is the first thing I do to stir up a storm?

3. **The Dead Weight:** If I were to be brutally honest, which habits, recurring thoughts, or "comfortable" relationships am I clinging to purely because they allow me to stay small and hidden?

4. **The Protection Tax:** What is my self-sabotage actually costing me? Not just in money or time, but in peace, sleep, and the person I promised my younger self I would become?

5. **The Permission Slip:** Whose approval am I still waiting for before I give myself permission to stop being a "mess" and start being a masterpiece?

The Final Reckoning

Let's be real: You've been carrying the weight of your past like it's a trophy. You're trying to tread water while clutching the very stones designed to sink you, and then you're wondering why you're drowning.

Here is the hard truth: **The door to your future is too narrow to fit you and all that baggage.**

That doorway wasn't built for the version of you that's still lugging around the armor, the excuses, and the "safety" of your self-sabotage. It was built for the person you were created to be. You have reached the point where you have to make a choice.

You can have your excuses, or you can have your **growth.** You cannot have both.

I know it's terrifying to let go. I know those stones feel like they belong to you. But your hands are so full of the past that you have no way to grab hold of tomorrow or even live today.

My question to you is: What are you finally ready to set down? What are you leaving on this page so your hands are finally free to build something new?

THE COMMMITMENT:
I Am Showing Up for Me

The Release: Emptying Your Hands

I want you to take a deep breath and be completely honest with yourself. What are you finally ready to let go of? Is it a habit that keeps you hidden? A lie that tells you you're not enough? Or a memory you use to punish yourself? I know it's scary to let go. You've clutched these things for so long that your hands feel cramped and tired. But you cannot reach for your future while your fingers are still locked around your past. You need to empty your hands so they are free to receive the good things that have been trying to find you all along.

Stop tripping yourself. You don't have to run a marathon today, and you don't need all the answers. You just have to stop tying your own feet together. Just one honest, shaky, real step forward. That is enough.

The Choice: A New Ground to Stand On

Now, look at those empty hands. It's time to make a promise to the person you are becoming. This isn't about being perfect; it's about being present. Say these words to yourself:

THE COMMITMENT:
I Am Showing Up for Me

Today, I'm done living on autopilot. I am choosing to finally look my habits in the eye instead of just letting them run my life. I'm trading the constant, screaming chaos for a single moment of quiet. I'm tired of the noise, and I'm tired of the fight.

I am done running from myself. I will no longer sprint away from my own heart; instead, I'm going to sit with my feelings, the good, the bad, and the ugly, and meet them with nothing but the raw truth. I don't have to hide anymore. I am finally safe enough to slow down. I am safe enough to let the healing actually touch the places that hurt. I am safe enough to grow.

With every breath I take, I am choosing my peace over my past. I am letting go of the person I had to be just to survive, and I am finally becoming the person I was meant to be.

Signed, _______________________________________

(No more excuses. No more waiting. This is who I am now.)

THE FINAL CHARGE:
You've Got the Power to Begin Again

Healing doesn't happen in the places where you've made yourself "comfortable" in your pain. It doesn't happen in the shadows where you've hidden your secrets. Healing only begins when you finally stop running and stand face-to-face with the truth.

I know the autopilot of self-sabotage feels like it's part of your DNA, but it's not. It's just a path you've walked so many times that your feet know the way by heart. Today, you are choosing a new trail.

Every time you catch yourself about to pull the trigger on a bad habit, and you pause, you are winning. Every time you choose awareness over autopilot, you are ripping up the old script and rewriting your story in real-time. You aren't that "mess" I used to see in the mirror. You are a person who is finally safe enough to respond instead of reacting.

You don't have to be perfect to be free. You just have to be willing to stop tripping yourself. The door is open, the path is clear, and for the first time in a long time, you are the one holding the keys.

Take the step. You are ready.

THE SEAL:
A Prayer for Your New Beginning

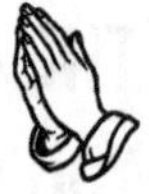

Dear Heavenly Father,
I'm being honest today: I've been my own worst enemy.
I've spent years building walls and calling them "safety,"
using my sabotage to keep the world at a distance. I
am tired of wearing a mask and tired of burning down
every good thing before it has a chance to grow.

Lord, help me drop these stones. My hands are
cramped from holding onto my past, and I'm exhausted
from trying to protect myself in my own power. I realize
now that I don't have to be strong enough to change
on my own. Your Word says I can do all things through
Christ who gives me strength, including the hard work
of letting go.

When the fear kicks in and I want to run back to the
chaos I know, steady my feet with Your power. Drown
out the old lies with Your truth and love. I'm stepping
out of the trenches today, choosing peace over my
past. I am letting go of the matches, trusting that
through Your strength, I can finally walk into the life
You have for me.

Thank You for being a God of new beginnings. I am choosing to believe that my future is not a repeat of my past. I am stepping out of the wreckage and into the light. I am letting go of the matches, and I am trusting You to lead the way.

In Jesus' Name,
Amen

*"I can do all this
through Him who gives me strength."*

— Philippians 4:13 NIV

My Notes

Date: ______________

My Notes

Date: _______________

My Notes

Date: _______________

My Notes

Date: ___________

CHAPTER 3

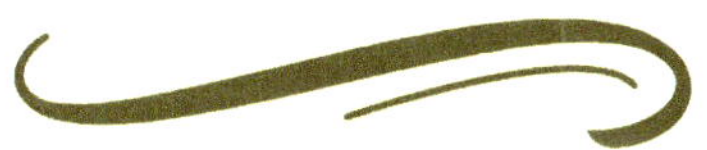

TAKE OFF THE MASK

The trade: real over "fine"

THE INVITATION:
Behind The Mask

Let's be real, "I'm fine" has become one of the biggest lies we tell. It's the mask we wear when we're breaking inside but don't want anyone to see. It's the shield we hide behind because admitting "I'm not okay" feels too risky. You've become so good at pretending that sometimes you even believe it. You've built a reputation for being strong, the one who holds it together, the one who keeps smiling. But what no one sees is that behind that mask, you're exhausted. Tired of holding it all in and carrying the weight of everyone else's expectations while silently falling apart.

MY STORY:
The Master of Disguise

The War Behind the Mask

I need you to lean in and really hear what I'm telling you: taking off my mask wasn't a casual choice. It was a battle for my life. For decades, the thought of letting anyone see the real me, the mess, the jagged pieces, the raw insecurity, was so terrifying that my anxiety would hit the roof just thinking about it.

I was raised on an unspoken rule: "Just deal with it." I was told early on that no one was listening, so I did the only thing I knew how to do, I silenced my own soul and buried the mess where I thought no one would find it. I became the "Queen of Excuses" and a master of disguise. If I could deflect you with a smile or a "perfect" answer, or with laughter. I knew you wouldn't see that I was actually bleeding out right in front of you.

The Midnight of the Soul

I reached a place so dark and so lonely that I didn't want to be in this world anymore. I'm not proud of that moment, but I am putting it on these pages because

I know some of you are sitting in that same darkness right as you read this. When you are at your lowest, giving up feels like the only exit left.

If you're sitting in that darkness right now, I need you to hear me: Giving up isn't the exit you think it is. It doesn't end the pain; it just passes the weight to the people who love you, leaving them with a void that can never be filled.

I thank God every single day that He stood in the gap for me. He didn't judge me for being tired, and He didn't turn away from my mess. Instead, He stood in the way of the door I was trying to close. He blocked my exit because He knew that my story, and yours, was never meant to end in the dark. He knew there were chapters ahead that I couldn't see yet. He knew that the world needed the version of me the one He created me to be, that was still to come.

I'm living proof that the darkness doesn't get the final word. My life wasn't over then, and I promise you, yours isn't over now. You aren't just surviving a tragedy; you are waiting for the dawn. Hold on. The light is coming.

The Weight of the Lie

To take off my mask, I had to face my greatest "protector": my pride. I didn't want anyone to see the real me because, honestly, I didn't even like the person I saw in the mirror. I realized my emotions were driving my life, but I finally had to admit that emotions are liars. They change with the wind and trick you into making decisions that betray your future.

I had become an expert at lying to the world, but the person I lied to most was myself. My mask had stopped being a shield and started being a lead weight, crushing me mentally, physically, and spiritually.

Choosing Life

I knew if I didn't change, I wouldn't survive the year. I had to tear down the walls of pride and finally, for the first time, reach out for help. I had to find the true Aroha, not for my mother, not for my *whānau or friends*, but for **me.**

It's time to stop the act. As you read these words, I want you to know it is okay to be done with the "I'm fine" lie. It's time to take off the mask and begin the messy, beautiful, life-saving journey of healing. You aren't "fine," and that's okay, because "fine" never healed anyone, but the truth will.

THE TRUTH:
"Fine" Is The Most Dangerous Lie

Take Off the Mask: The Trade

Let's stop the games. **"I'm fine" is the most dangerous lie you tell.** You wear that mask because you're terrified that your real mess is too much for the world to handle. You've convinced yourself that if you show the jagged edges or the parts of you that are actually screaming, you'll be met with judgment or pity. So, you choose the "safe" route: you stay busy, you keep smiling, and you perform "strength" while you're bleeding out internally.

But here is the brutal truth: You cannot heal a person you refuse to be.

You are exhausting yourself trying to protect a version of you that doesn't even exist. You think this fake strength is your shield, but it's actually your cage. You've let your pain move into your heart, unpack its bags, and start making the rules. But pain was only ever meant to be a teacher. It was supposed to show you where you were broken so you could find a cure; it was never meant to be the tenant that owns your soul.

Stop Performing for a God Who Already Sees You

Why are you still trying to hide from the only One who already knows your secrets? God meets you in your truth, not your performance. He isn't looking for a polished version of your story. He doesn't want the "Sunday morning" mask or the "strong warrior" act.

He cannot heal a mask. He won't fix a fake. He is waiting for the real you, the one who is tired, messy, and scared, to finally step out of the shadows. You are choosing to stay sick just so you can stay "private." Is your pride really worth your life?

The Challenge: Let it Fall

This is your permission slip to stop the act. You don't have to have it all together to be worthy of love. You don't have to be "fixed" to be saved. You just have to be real.

The moment you stop performing is the moment you can finally catch your breath. Take off the mask. It's heavy, it's suffocating, and it's lying to you every single day. The truth will feel shaky and raw at first, but it is the only ground solid enough to build a new home on.

The trade is simple, but it's a battle: Give up the "fine" lie today, or stay trapped in it forever. Which one do you want more?

THE REALITY CHECK: Your Brain is is an Overprotective Bodyguard

We need to talk about why you can't seem to stop pretending. Your brain isn't trying to make you miserable; it's just obsessed with keeping you **safe.**

Somewhere in your past, being "real" got you hurt. Maybe you were mocked, ignored, or told to "just get over it." Your brain took a mental snapshot of that pain and made a vow: *"Never again."* From that day on, it began building your mask. It convinced you that "I'm fine" was the only way to survive the room you were in.

The Cage of Strength

Your brain treats vulnerability like a death threat. When you even think about being honest, your nervous system sounds the alarm and hits panic mode. That spike in anxiety, the lump in your throat, the urge to run, that is your internal bodyguard trying to force the armor back on. It thinks the mask is your only shield.

But here is the truth your brain doesn't understand: The armor that kept you safe back then is the cage that is destroying you now. You aren't tired from doing too much; you are tired from hiding too much. Every time you bury your truth, you aren't deleting it, you're just pressurizing it. Eventually, it will leak out through anger, burnout, or a numbness that leaves you feeling like a ghost in your own life.

The Challenge: Rewire for Truth

Honesty won't break you; it's the only thing that will finally allow your nervous system to rest. You have to prove to your brain that you are safe enough to be real. When the alarm goes off and you feel the urge to hide behind "I'm fine," stop. Don't fight the bodyguard, just quiet him down.

THE DRILL:
Finding Your Breath in the Storm (The Honesty Practice)

After years of hiding, being seen can feel scary. This practice helps you break the habit of "I'm Fine" and teaches your mind that being real makes you free:

1. **Notice When You Shrink:** Pay attention to the moments you go quiet, change the subject, or instinctively say "I'm fine." Don't judge the response, just acknowledge it.

2. **Ask What You're Scared Of:** When you catch yourself hiding, gently ask: "What am I afraid people will see if I stop pretending?" Naming the fear removes its power.

3. **Tell One Small Truth:** You don't need to spill everything. Say to a safe person, "Actually, today's been a bit hard," or "I'm trying to figure things out."

4. **Stand in Your Truth:** Don't rush to laugh it off or take it back. Let the truth stay.

5. **Rebuild Trust with Yourself:** Make and keep one small promise to yourself today (e.g., *I will rest for 15 minutes, I will say no to one request*).

The 30-Second Reset: "The Truth Breath"

When you feel the mask trying to slide back on, or your chest starts to tighten, do this immediately to signal "safety" to your brain:

1. **Exhale first:** Blow all the air out of your mouth like you're blowing through a straw. Get to the very bottom of the breath.

2. **The Inhale (4 seconds):** Breathe in slowly through your nose, imagining you are breathing in the word **"Grace."**

3. **The Hold (4 seconds):** Hold that breath. Tell your brain: "I am safe to be seen."

4. **The Release (6 seconds):** Exhale even slower than you inhaled, imagining you are dropping the weight of the word **"Fine."**

THE HARD QUESTIONS:
What Are You Tired of Carrying?

Be honest, even if it stings. Healing is impossible if you keep pretending you don't see the wreckage in front of you. Take a breath, grab a pen, and look at the truth.

1. **What is the "I'm fine" lie actually covering up today?** If you stripped away the smile and the "perfect" answer, what would be left? Is it a fear that you're failing? Is it a deep, quiet loneliness? Or is it a mountain of grief you've never been allowed to cry over? Don't give the "polite" answer, give the real one.

2. **What has the "cost of admission" been for your mask?** Pretending isn't free; it's the most expensive thing you own. Look at your life, what has it cost you? Has it cost you your sleep? Your ability to feel real joy? Has it created a wall between you and the people who actually love you? Write down exactly what this mask has stolen from your soul.

3. **What is the worst thing you think would happen if you said, "Actually, I'm not okay"?** Trace that fear to the end. Do you think you'll be rejected? Do you think the world will fall apart if you aren't the

one holding it up? Now, ask yourself: *Is that the truth, or is that just my "bodyguard" brain trying to keep me hidden?*

4. **Who would you be if you didn't have to be "strong" anymore?** Imagine a version of yourself that didn't have to perform, deflect, or hide. If you didn't have to carry everyone else's expectations, what would you do with all that extra energy? Who is the person underneath all that armor?

THE COMMMITMENT:
I Am Showing Up for Me

Today, I am making a decision that my past no longer has the right to dictate my future. I am resigning from the role of the "perfect" one and the "master of disguise." I am done using excuses to hide my heart. I am finally showing up for myself, and for today, that is enough.

I no longer hide behind the mask of "I'm fine." I recognize that "fine" has become my prison, and I am choosing the keys of truth to let myself out. I choose the raw reality of my life over the polished lie of my performance. I am learning to trust my own voice again, even if it shakes, one honest word at a time.

I am safe to be seen. I silence the lies of my overprotective brain that tell me vulnerability is a death sentence. I am safe to be loved in my mess, and I am safe to grow in my brokenness. I realize now that my true strength isn't found in how much I can carry alone; my strength is found in my honesty, and my power is found in my peace.

I release the need to perform. I don't have to earn my place in this world, and I don't have to be "together" to be worthy of grace. I am trading my heavy armor for a life of freedom. I am stepping out of the shadows and into the light of the person I was always meant to be.

Signed, ____

(No more excuses. No more waiting. This is who I am now.)

THE FINAL CHARGE:
You've Got the Power to Begin Again

Stop Hiding the Hurt

Listen to me: you cannot heal while you are still hiding. You can't walk into your future if you are still trying to live as a version of yourself that isn't real. Taking off the mask doesn't mean you are weak; it means you finally care enough about yourself to stop pretending. You can't find true peace while you are still putting on a performance.

Choose Real Over "Fine"

You've been wearing this disguise for too long, just trying to make it through the day. But you were made for more than just "getting by." You were made to be known and to be whole. Choosing to be real is how the healing finally starts. If you don't let the act go, the pressure of being "fine" will eventually be the only thing you feel. It's time to trade the fake smile for the honest truth.

Make Room for Peace

Here is a hard truth: you cannot be helped if you won't be seen. If your hands are busy holding up a mask of "perfection" or "strength," there is no room for the genuine joy and rest that is waiting for you. You are blocking your own path to freedom by refusing to show your real face.

End the Act

Let it fall. All of it. The "I'm fine" lie, the excuses, and the walls you built to stay safe. You were never meant to live in a cage of your own making, and you don't have to stay there for one more minute. You aren't waiting for a miracle, you are the one holding the key to the door.

The power to start over isn't in someone else's hands; it's in yours. Open your hands. Let the mask hit the ground. Take your first breath as a real, free person.

THE SEAL:
A Prayer for the Real Me

Dear Heavenly Father,

You see who I really am when I'm all alone. You know how much energy I've spent trying to look like I have it all together, and you know how tired I am of the act. You've seen me play the part and hide my pain, even when I felt like I was breaking inside.

Today, I'm done with the disguise. I'm trading the heavy weight of my pride for the freedom of being real. I'm finished silencing my own heart just to make everyone else feel comfortable. I'm stepping out from behind the curtain.

Please give me the courage to be honest, even when it feels scary. Help me see that being "real" is so much better than being "fine." Give me the wisdom to know when people are taking advantage of my kindness, and the strength to say "no" so I can stay whole.

I'm letting the mask fall to the floor. I choose to believe that I am enough without the performance. I trust that the real me, the one without the excuses and the fake smiles, is the only one who can truly heal.

The act is over. The mask is gone. I'm finally choosing to step into the light.

In Jesus' Name,

Amen

*"Then you will know the truth,
and the truth will set you free."*

— John 8:32 NIV

My Notes

Date: ___________________

My Notes

Date: _______________

My Notes

Date: _______________

My Notes

Date: _______________

PART TWO

Reclaim

The Internal Reset:
Taking Back the Ground You Lost

CHAPTER 4

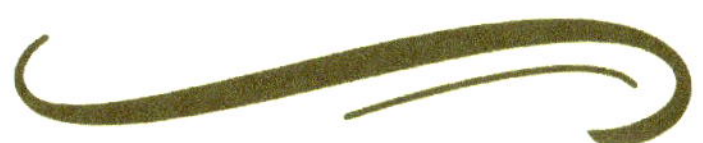

PUT DOWN THE STONES

Evict the bitterness. Drop the weight.

THE INVITATION:
Letting Go

One of the hardest things you'll ever do is letting go. You tell yourself you've moved on, but deep down, the hurt still lingers in the dark corners of your heart. You replay the moments, the words, and the actions until the pain feels like a shadow following you everywhere you go. It changes how you trust, how you think, and how you see the world. Anger begins to grow, and you wonder why you should forgive when they were the ones who caused the damage. You try to let it go, but your chest still tightens every time their name comes up. I need you to hear me: holding on doesn't protect you; it is draining the very life out of you.

MY STORY:
Survival, A Badge Of Honor

The War Behind Dropping the Weight

For a long time, I wore my survival like a badge of honor, but underneath the surface, I was suffocating. I carried wounds I never asked for, rejection that stung like ice, emotional abuse that eroded my confidence, and sexual abuse that tried to steal my very soul. These weren't just memories; they were stones I carried in my pockets every single day. I thought that keeping them, holding onto the weight of what was done to me, was a form of strength. I thought if I stayed angry enough, or blocked it out, I was staying safe. But the truth was, I was just exhausted. I was the "Queen of Being Okay," while secretly I was wondering why I was the one left to clean up a mess I didn't make.

The Midnight of the Soul

There were nights when the weight of those stones felt like they were dragging me to the bottom of an ocean. I would sit in the wreckage of my past and look at the people who hurt me, people who were out living their lives, untouched by the damage they left behind, while I was paralyzed by the bill they ran up. It felt permanent. It felt like pain had signed a lifelong lease on my heart and changed the locks. I didn't just feel hurt; I felt haunted. I reached a point where I couldn't see a future because the past was taking up all the room.

The Divine Gap

In that darkness, I heard a whisper that shifted everything: *"You are holding onto the stones that were meant to be thrown at you, but I have already stepped in front of them."* I realized that God wasn't asking me to ignore what happened, but He was standing in the door to my past so I could finally turn around and see my future. He showed me that while I didn't start the fire, I didn't have to keep standing in the ashes. He stood in the gap between the girl who was broken and the woman He was calling me to be, reminding me that the "mess" was never my identity, it was just the location where He found me. It was time to let go of the stones of bitterness, anger and hatred.

THE TRUTH:
Forgiveness Is Your Freedom

The Heavy Reality

Let's be honest with ourselves. Unforgiveness isn't just a feeling; it's a heavy backpack full of jagged stones that cuts into your soul every single day. Every "why" that keeps you awake at night, every bit of resentment you hold onto, it's just more weight. You're exhausted because you're trying to move forward while carrying the very things that were meant to keep you down. You've been carrying this for so long that you've forgotten what it feels like to walk light and free.

Forgiveness is Your Freedom

We need to get one thing straight: Forgiveness does NOT mean what they did was okay. It doesn't mean they get a pass for the damage they caused. It means: "You don't get to control my peace for one more second." It's a firm, quiet choice to choose your own life over the desire to stay stuck in the hurt. Holding onto the pain is like staying in a cage with the person who hurt you. Forgiveness is you finally turning the key, walking out the door, and choosing never to look back. It's not about them; it's about you refusing to be a prisoner to your past.

The Awareness of Grace

As you walk toward that door, you have to be careful. We are taught to offer grace, but we must also be aware of what I call the abuse of grace. There is a difference between a person who is truly sorry for their behavior and a person who uses your kindness or vulnerability as a doormat for their own personal gain. Some will expect your forgiveness to be a blank check for their toxicity, returning to the same hurtful patterns like a dog returning to its own vomit. They aren't looking for a change of heart; they are looking for control. You must realize that grace is not a permission slip for your own destruction. You can forgive someone and still keep the door locked. You can release the debt without letting them back into your space to hurt you again. True peace cannot be found in a place where you are constantly being hunted by someone else's choices or control.

The Hourly Choice

Forgiveness isn't a one-time event; it's a choice you make over and over again. Most days, it's an hourly decision to stay free. It's that moment when the old hurt starts to rise up in your chest and you have to tell yourself: "No. I'm not going back there. You don't live here anymore." It's learning to capture the toxic thoughts that no longer deserve to be the ruler of your mind let alone your life. It's learning to speak the truth over you with love and compassion. Your pain was meant to be a teacher, it was meant to show you your boundaries and how strong you truly are. But somewhere along the way, you let it move in. You let it become a tenant in a heart that belongs to you.

Release the Weight

It's time to stop hosting the things that are trying to break you. That weight you're dragging around? It has overstayed its welcome. You don't have to carry that backpack for one more step. You can set it down right here, on this page, and just keep walking. Your future is waiting, and it's beautiful, but you need your hands empty to reach for it.

Drop the weight. Take your peace back. You have a life to live, and you deserve to breathe again.

THE REALITY CHECK:
Your Brain Needs A New Compass

The Familiar Ache

You can't control what broke you, but you have every right to control how long you let it live inside your head. We often wait for a "feeling" of peace before we decide to let go, but let's be real: if you wait until letting go feels "good," you'll be waiting forever. Your brain holds onto old pain and replays those jagged memories because it mistakes that familiar ache for safety. It's a survival instinct. Your mind thinks that by keeping the hurt close, it's keeping you on high alert so you never get caught off guard again.

The False Alarm

Hear me clearly: your brain isn't trying to punish you; it's trying to protect you. It's scanning the horizon for the next threat, using your past trauma as a map. This is why choosing to forgive and move forward feels so incredibly uncomfortable, it's not what your used to. Your brain sees the "peace" you're searching for as a "danger zone" because it's unfamiliar territory. But just because a feeling is familiar doesn't mean it's healthy, and just because a new path feels scary doesn't mean you're in danger. It just means you're finally growing beyond the walls of your cage.

Reclaiming Your Space

Forgiveness isn't about the person who caused the pain, it's about the person who has to live with it. It's not a reward for their bad behavior; it's an act of self-rescue for your future, for your peace. You are simply deciding that your mental real estate is too precious to be rented out to people who only bring storms and drama. It's you stepping up and telling your survival instincts, "I appreciate you looking out for me, but I'm taking my power back now.

The New Compass

It's time to rewire the way you navigate your life. You've been using your wounds as a compass for too long, and they've only ever led you back to the same dark places. You have to be brave enough to be uncomfortable for a little while as you learn to walk without the weight of that high alert. You aren't "losing your guard"; you are finally finding your peace.

Stop letting your survival instincts steal your future. Your brain is trying to keep you safe, but God is trying to keep you whole.

THE DRILL:
The Hands-Open Release
(Freedom Practice)

When bitterness and old hurts take up space in your heart, they manifest as physical tension. Your hands clench, your shoulders rise, and your heart feels heavy. This practice is designed to help you physically and mentally "drop the stones" and train your brain to let go.

1. **Find the Physical Weight.** Sit quietly and notice where you are holding tension. Are your fists clenched? Is your jaw tight? This physical "grip" is often a reflection of the emotional stones you are still carrying.

2. **The "Stonework" Visualization.** Close your eyes and imagine the person or situation you are bitter toward. Visualize that hurt as a heavy, jagged stone in each of your hands. Feel the weight. Notice how much energy it takes just to keep holding on.

3. **The Exhale Eviction.** Take a deep breath in through your nose. As you breathe out slowly through your mouth, physically open your hands wide. Imagine those stones falling away. Say quietly: "I am no longer a storage unit for this pain."

4. **Name the Release.** Specifically name what you are dropping. Say: "I am dropping the stone of [*Name of Hurt/Person*]. It is no longer mine to carry."

5. **Claim the Empty Space.** Rest with your palms facing upward. Do not rush to fill the void. Tell your brain: "My hands are empty so they can finally be open to something new."

THE HARD QUESTIONS:
What Are You Tired of Carrying?

I want you to take a deep breath and just be still for a second. We've talked about the weight and the stones, but now I want to look at your hands. Healing doesn't happen until we stop hiding from ourselves. I'm going to ask you a few simple questions. Don't rush to answer them with your head, listen to what your heart says. Be honest, even if it's a little uncomfortable.

1. **What am I actually afraid will happen if I let this go?** Are you worried that if you stop being angry, you'll be left unprotected? Do you feel like your pain is the only thing keeping you safe from being hurt again? Ask yourself if you've been using your hurt as a wall, and if you're scared of what life looks like without that wall to hide behind.

2. **Am I still waiting for an apology that is never going to come?** Is there a part of you that feels like you can't move on until they admit they were wrong? I want to be honest with you. Most likely you will never receive an apology. When we wait for someone else to say "I'm sorry" before we find our peace, we are giving them the remote control to our lives. Are you okay with letting the person who hurt you decide when you get to be happy?

3. **What could I do with my life if I wasn't so tired from carrying this?** Think about all the energy you spend thinking about the past, replaying the hurt, and managing your anger. If you could have all that energy back today, what would you do with it? If your hands were finally empty, what beautiful thing would you reach for instead?

4. **Am I mistaking "being a good person" for being a doormat?** Are you holding onto this because you think *grace* means you have to keep taking the hits? Are you staying silent just to keep a "peace" that isn't actually peaceful for you? Ask yourself if you are protecting someone else's reputation at the expense of your own soul.

THE COMMMITMENT:
I Am Showing Up for Me

Healing is not an accident; it is a choice. It's time to stop waiting for the weight to fall off and start choosing to set it down. I want you to say these words out loud, not because they are "magic," but because your soul needs to hear your own voice claiming its freedom.

Healing is not an accident; it is a choice.

I Am Not My Past

I am not the things that happened to me, and I am not the mistakes I made while I was trying to survive. My history is a part of my journey, but it is not my identity. I am the one who survived, and I am the one who gets to decide what happens next.

I Release the Weight

I am done being a storage unit for other people's toxic choices. I release what was never mine to carry. I am handing back the shame, the guilt, and the "why" that belongs to someone else. My hands are becoming empty so they can finally be open.

I Surrender the Hurt

I forgive what I cannot change, and I surrender the parts of me that still ache. I'm not waiting for an apology to be okay. I am choosing peace over anger, and I am choosing grace over bitterness. I am no longer a doormat; I am a person of worth with boundaries that protect my soul.

I Walk in Freedom

Today, I am choosing my own life. I am walking away from the heavy weight of the past and stepping into the light. For the first time, I am showing up for myself, the real me. I'm doing it without the mask, without the baggage, and without the lies.

I'm not pretending anymore. I'm finally free.

Today, I walk in forgiveness. Today, I walk in freedom. Today, I am coming home to myself.

Signed, ____
(No more excuses. No more waiting. This is who I am now.)

THE FINAL CHARGE:
You've Got the Power to Begin Again

The Danger of the Silence

The moment you truly drop the stones, something terrifying happens: it gets quiet. For years, your bitterness gave you a purpose. It gave you something to talk about, something to obsess over, and a reason to stay guarded. When you finally evict the bitterness, you are left with a void. This is the "danger zone." Most people pick their stones back up not because they want the pain, but because they can't handle the emptiness. They don't know who they are without their grudge.

Don't Fill the Space with Junk

You have just cleared out the "mental real estate" that was being occupied by your past. Now, you have to be the intentional architect of what goes there next. If you don't intentionally fill those empty hands with something new, a new passion, a new boundary, or a new mission, you will instinctively reach back for the weight of your old resentment just to feel "full" again.

From Carrying Weight to Using Strength

Moving forward isn't just about what you *stopped* doing. It's about what you're going to do with all that extra energy. You used to spend so much of yourself just managing your anger and holding onto those stones. Now, that energy is yours again. The question is no longer "Why did they hurt me?" The question is now "What am I going to do with the strength I used to waste on them?"

THE SEAL:
A Prayer for Your New Beginning

Dear Heavenly Father,

You know the parts of me that still ache. Today, I choose to surrender them to You. I let go of what's behind me and I trust You with what's ahead. Teach me to stop picking up what I've already laid at Your feet. Fill me with peace where pain used to live. I choose to live lighter, freer, and closer to You.

In Jesus' Name,
Amen

"Come to me, all you who are weary and burdened, and I will give you rest."

— *Matthew 11:28* NIV

My Notes

Date: _______________

My Notes

Date: ___________________

My Notes

Date: ____________________

My Notes

Date: ___________________

CHAPTER 5

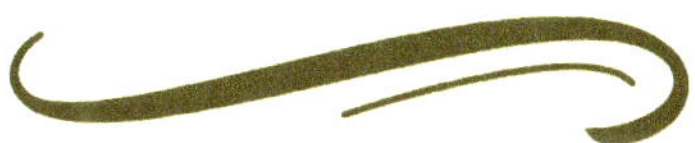

THE INTERNAL RESET

Aligning your mind to stop the cycle of failure

THE INVITATION:
Ending the Internal Conflict

You are standing at a crossroads.

Your hands are empty, but your mind is still clenched. You have dropped the stones, but your body is still braced for the weight. This is the "Phantom Burden", the moment where the freedom you prayed for starts to feel like a threat.

If you don't choose a new direction, your brain will trick you into picking your old pain back up just to feel "normal" again.

I am inviting you to stop the "Failure Stack." It is time to end the internal tug-of-war between the heart that is ready to fly and the brain that is terrified of the heights. In this next chapter, we will align your mind with your vision so you can stop sabotaging your peace and start building your future.

The cage is open. Now, let's learn how to walk through it.

MY STORY:
The Internal Tug-of-War

If you are like me, you've had the best intentions. You've set the goals, read the books, avoided the toxic people, and maybe even sat through the classes or started a new job. You had the toolkit ready to go. But then, the old habits started whispering. They didn't just whisper; they screamed, reminding you of exactly who you used to be.

In my journey of learning to let go of the pain, I realized something brutal: Freedom isn't a straight line.

I felt like I was in a constant battle for my own attention. On one side was the person I wanted to become; on the other was the person I had been for years. I was an expert at cataloging my flaws. Every time I tried to make a better choice, I'd find myself back in a toxic environment or around the wrong people, and—*snap*—I'd slip. The walls went up. The "talk to the hand" expression returned. The anger flared.

I was retreating to the only "comfort zone" I knew: toxicity. And every time I slipped, I felt worse than before. That is exactly what **Failure Stacking** looks like. You take one bad moment and use it as a brick to rebuild your old prison.

I finally reached a breaking point where I realized I had nothing left to lose, but everything to gain by stepping into the uncomfortable "growth zone." I had to accept a hard truth: this wasn't going to happen overnight. I had to stop wishing for a miracle and start making intentional decisions. I had to ask myself: *Was I going to let one mistake define me, or was I going to dust myself off and start fresh every single time?*

I learned that every hurdle wasn't a stop sign; it was a weight-lifting session. It gave me the strength to keep moving. I learned how to intercept the toxic thoughts before they hit the ground and replace them with something better.

So, let me be raw with you: **don't beat yourself up when you stumble.** You will fall. Expect it. But don't let a fall become a "stack." Just like a professional athlete, you don't quit the game because you missed one shot. You acknowledge the miss, adjust your aim, and get back on the court. You have a goal ahead of you, don't let a temporary trip keep you from a permanent destination.

THE TRUTH:
The Basic Truths of the Reset

1. **Your Brain is a Creature of Habit, Not Truth**
   Your brain doesn't care if a thought is "true" or "good" for you; it only cares if the thought is familiar. If you have been told you are a failure for twenty years, your brain thinks that is "home." When you try to be better, your brain feels "homesick" for the struggle.

   - **The Truth:** Feeling the urge to go back to your old ways isn't a sign that you haven't changed, it's just your brain's autopilot trying to stay in a familiar lane.

2. **You Cannot Build a New House with Old Trash**
   You cannot create a life of purpose if you are still using your past mistakes as your building materials. Every time you "Failure Stack," you are trying to build your future using the "trash" from your past.

   - **The Truth:** To reset, you have to stop looking at your past as a "description" of who you are and start seeing it as a "location" you used to live in. You don't live there anymore.

3. **Alignment is a Choice, Not a Feeling**
   You will not always *feel* aligned. There will be days
   your heart wants to grow but your brain is tired
   and cranky. If you wait until you "feel" like doing
   the right thing, you will never move.

   - **The Truth:** Alignment happens when you tell
     your brain what to do, rather than letting your
     brain tell you how to feel. You are the boss of
     your mind, not the other way around.

THE REALITY CHECK:
Getting Your Head and Heart on the Same Page

You stop the cycle of failure by giving your brain a new job. Instead of letting it look for mistakes, you train it to look for progress.

1. **Facts Over Feelings** Your heart is emotional. When you make a mistake, your heart feels like the world is ending. This is when you need to use your brain for facts.

   - **The simple shift:** When you mess up, stop and tell yourself: "This is just one mistake. It is not who I am." Don't let a feeling turn into a fact.

2. **Start Stacking Wins** Your brain believes whatever has the most "proof." Right now, it has a lot of proof of your past mistakes. You need to start giving it proof of your new life.

   - **The simple shift:** Every night, think of three small things you did right. Maybe you stayed calm, maybe you said "no" to a toxic thought or person, or maybe you just got out of bed. These are your new "bricks." You are building a new stack of wins.

3. **The Five-Second Reset** Your brain loves your "comfort zone," even if that zone is toxic. When you feel yourself getting angry or shutting down, you have about five seconds to stop it before your brain goes on autopilot.

   - **The simple shift:** The moment you feel that old "toxic" feeling, **move.** Stand up, drink some water, or take three deep breaths. This "resets" your brain and gives your heart a chance to choose a better reaction.

The Goal

When you align your heart and brain, you stop fighting yourself. You aren't just "trying" to be better; you are training yourself to be better. You are moving from a life of accidents to a life of purpose.

THE DRILL:
Your Daily Reset

When you make a mistake or feel a toxic thought coming on, don't panic. Just follow these three simple steps to stop the "failure stack" before it starts.

Step 1: The "Stop Sign" The second you realize you've messed up or stayed in a bad mood too long, you have to hit the brakes.

- **What to do:** Say to yourself, "That was a bad moment, but it's not a bad life."

- **Why it works:** This keeps the mistake small. It prevents one little slip-up from turning into a giant mountain of "proof" that you'll never change.

Step 2: The "Win Hunt" Your brain is naturally looking for what went wrong. You have to force it to look for what went right.

- **What to do:** Name one good thing you've done today. It can be as small as drinking enough water or choosing to be kind to a stranger.

- **Why it works:** This gives your brain "New Evidence." You are proving to your mind that you are making progress, even if it's just one inch at a time.

Step 3: The "Next Right Move" Don't worry about next week or even tonight. Just focus on the very next thing you need to do.

- **What to do:** Ask yourself, "What is the next right thing for the person I want to be?" Maybe it's taking a walk, finishing a task, or simply taking a deep breath.

- **Why it works:** This gets your brain out of the past and into the present. It puts you back in the driver's seat.

Practice Makes Permanent

You don't have to do this perfectly; you just have to do it consistently. Every time you use this drill, you are teaching your heart and brain how to work as a team. You are building a new habit of **success** instead of a habit of **failure.**

THE DISCOVERY QUESTIONS

Instead of looking at what's holding you back, let's look at how much room you have to grow. Answer these with kindness toward yourself.

1. **What does my "Peace" look like?** Instead of thinking about your toxic comfort zone, imagine your "Comfort Zone of Peace." When you feel completely aligned and calm, what are you doing? How does it feel to know that this version of you is the **real** you?

2. **What is my newest "Win"?** Think about one time recently, no matter how small, where you chose a good thought over a bad one. How can you use that one "brick" of success to start building a brand-new stack today?

3. **What is my heart's favorite truth?** Your brain might whisper lies, but your heart knows the truth. What is one positive thing you believe about your future? If that truth was the only thing guiding you today, what would your next step be?

You've Got This

Answering these questions isn't about digging up the past; it's about planting seeds for your future. You are no longer defined by the stack of what went wrong. You are defined by the direction you are walking in right now.

THE COMMMITMENT: A New Agreement

It is time to end the tug-of-war. Before you turn the page, take a moment to read this out loud. This is your "Internal Reset", a simple agreement to treat yourself with the same kindness and hope you give to others.

The Promise

- ***I choose to believe*** *that my mistakes are just lessons, not my identity.*

- ***I choose to notice*** *my small wins and stack them high.*

- ***I choose to listen*** *to my heart's vision instead of my brain's old fears.*

- ***I choose to start fresh*** *every single time I stumble, because my future is worth the effort.*

Signed, _______________________________________

(No more excuses. No more waiting. This is who I am now.)

THE FINAL CHARGE:

One Last Thought

You aren't just "trying" to change anymore. You are training your mind to see the goodness that was always there. The stones are gone, and the "phantom weight" is fading. You are standing tall, you are aligned, and you are ready for the purpose that has been waiting for you all along.

Take a deep breath. You are no longer stacking failures, you are building a life.

THE SEAL:
A Prayer for Alignment

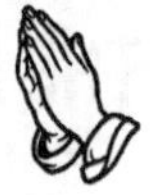

Dear Heavenly Father,

I thank You for this moment of reset. Thank You for the freedom of empty hands and the hope of a clear mind. Right now, I ask for Your help in ending the conflict within me.

Lord, when my brain tries to pull me back into old habits or remind me of past mistakes, help me to hear Your voice instead. When I feel the urge to "stack" my failures, remind me that Your mercies are new every single morning. Align my heart with Your vision for my life and settle my mind with Your peace.

Help me to see my progress, no matter how small. Give me the strength to dust myself off whenever I stumble and the courage to keep walking toward the future You have prepared for me. I am no longer a prisoner of my past; I am a child of Your purpose.

I choose to stand tall, to breathe deep, and to trust that You are building something beautiful in me, one win at a time.

In Jesus' Name,
Amen

*"Finally, brothers and sisters, whatever is true,
whatever is noble, whatever is right,
whatever is pure, whatever is lovely,
whatever is admirable, if anything is excellent
or praiseworthy, think about such things."*

Philippians 4:8 NKJV

My Notes

Date: ___________________

My Notes

Date: _______________

My Notes

Date: _______________

My Notes

Date: ___________

CHAPTER 6

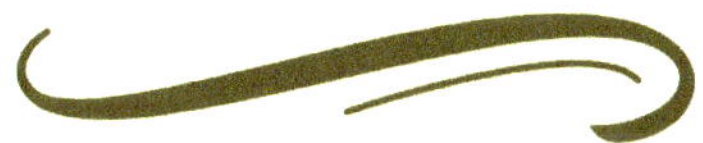

TRUSTING THE ONE IN THE MIRROR

The quiet inner strength of saying "no"

THE INVITATION:
The quiet inner strength in saying no

You have spent a lifetime trying to be "enough" for everyone else. You have kept your promises to your boss, your friends, and your family, but you have consistently broken the promises you made to yourself.

Every time you say "yes" to someone else when your heart is screaming "no," you lose a little bit of trust in the person looking back at you in the mirror. You feel shaky because you don't know if you can rely on yourself.

This chapter is your turning point.

We aren't going to build a loud, aggressive ego. Instead, we are going to build a quiet inner strength.

We are going to learn that saying **"no"** isn't an act of war, it's an act of honesty. It is the only way to protect the peace you've worked so hard to find.

It's time to stop looking for someone else to validate you and start becoming someone you can finally trust.

MY STORY:
The Cost of a "Yes"

For a long time, saying "no" to friends, family, or even strangers was the hardest thing for me to do. Why? Because I was a people pleaser. I didn't want to rock the boat or be the cause of any drama. I wanted to fit in, and I didn't care if it came at the expense of my own peace.

I knew the moment I said "yes" to something I should have declined. I could feel the pressure and weight start to build immediately. Then, panic mode would set in. I had no one else to blame but myself.

Does that sound familiar? Often, we are our own worst enemies. Nothing good ever came from my people-pleasing. I would pretend everything was fine on the outside, but inside, I was screaming: "Why did you say yes? Now you have to live with the consequences." I didn't learn my lesson right away, either. I repeatedly said "yes" to my own detriment until my body started to pay the price. The emotional pain turned into physical sickness, stress, and mental exhaustion. I was trying to "keep up with the Joneses," but that path only leads to one place: total burnout. I was exhausted from trying to maintain the lie that "everything is okay."

The Turning Point

It took a while, but I finally started to say "no." I began with the little things. As I gained confidence and realized the crushing pressure was disappearing, I began to extend that "no" to bigger requests, things that were beyond my capability or simply weren't healthy for me or my family.

As time went on, my confidence grew. I realized that by saying "no" to the wrong things, I finally had the time and energy to say **"YES"** to the things that actually mattered.

The word **"No"** became so powerful that I stopped allowing people to use me as a doormat. Today, I have no problem saying "no" to anything that isn't good for my soul or my family.

My Encouragement to You

I want to encourage you: start small. As you begin to say "no," you will gain confidence, strength, and, believe it or not, wisdom. I learned that saying "no" is the ultimate way to protect your inner peace. Learning this was one of the most transforming and freeing moments of my life.

THE TRUTH:
Ending the Internal Lie

The hardest part about being a people-pleaser is that it forces you to live a lie. Every time you smile and say, "Sure, I can do that," while your heart is sinking, you are being dishonest with yourself and the person standing in front of you.

The truth is simple: You cannot give what you do not have.

If you are running on empty, saying "yes" doesn't make you a better person, it just makes you a resentful one. True inner strength starts with the courage to be honest about your limits.

- **Honesty over Harmony:** We often choose "harmony" (not rocking the boat) over "honesty." But harmony built on a lie isn't real peace; it's just a temporary truce.

- **The Weight of the Mask:** It is exhausting to pretend you are okay when you are burnt out. The moment you speak your truth and say "no," the mask falls off, and for the first time in a long time, you can actually breathe.

- **Respect Follows Truth:** Ironically, people don't truly respect a doormat; they respect someone who knows their value. When you start speaking the truth about what you can and cannot do, the world begins to see you differently because you see yourself differently.

The Mirror Check

Stand in front of the mirror and look yourself in the eyes. Ask yourself: "Am I being honest with my 'Yes,' or am I just afraid of the conflict a 'No' might bring?" The truth might feel uncomfortable at first, but it is the only thing that will set you free from the cycle of burnout. You aren't "letting people down" by being honest; you are finally standing up for the life you were meant to live.

THE REALITY CHECK:
Small Wins, Real Trust

The reality is that you don't need a massive life overhaul to find your strength. You just need to stop breaking the small promises you make to yourself. Trust is built like a brick wall, one small, honest action at a time.

Here are three realistic ways to start rebuilding that trust today.

The Three Steps to Self-Trust

1. **The "Power of One" Promise:** Don't try to change your whole routine. Just pick one thing you will do for yourself today and stick to it, no matter what.

    - **The Goal:** It could be as simple as making your bed as soon as you get up, or taking a ten-minute walk.

    - **Why it works:** When you follow through on this one small thing, you prove to the person in the mirror that you are reliable.

2. **The Five-Second Pause:** We often say "yes" to people before we even think about it.

    - **The Goal:** The next time someone asks you for a favor or your time, wait five seconds before answering.

    - **Why it works:** That tiny pause gives you the space to ask yourself: "Do I actually want to do this?" It prevents you from making a promise you'll later regret or resent.

3. **Set a "Quiet Time":** Choose a 30-minute window today where you are "off-duty" from everyone else's needs.

    - **The Goal:** Turn off your notifications or go to a quiet room. Use this time to just be still or do something you enjoy.

    - **Why it works:** Keeping this appointment with yourself shows that your time has value. You are teaching yourself that you are worth the same respect you give to others.

The 24-Hour Challenge

For the next 24 hours, focus on being **100% honest** with your commitments. If you don't want to do something, don't say "maybe" or "later", just say "I'm not able to do that."

The Goal: End your day knowing you didn't over-commit. Experience the relief of having a schedule that actually belongs to you. This is where your new strength begins.

THE DRILL:
Protecting Your Reset

Now that you have the tools, it's time to put them into practice. People around you are used to the "old you", the one who always said yes. When you start saying no, they might push back. This drill is designed to help you hold your ground without losing your peace.

1. **The "Broken Record" Technique**

    When you say no, people will often ask "Why?" or try to talk you into it. You don't need a better excuse; you just need to repeat your truth.

    - **The Drill:** Practice saying a simple phrase like: "I understand, but I'm just not able to commit to that right now."

    - **The Challenge:** If they ask again, repeat the exact same sentence. Don't add more details. Eventually, they will realize your "No" is firm.

2. **The Notification Lockdown**

    Your phone is a door that anyone can walk through at any time. To protect your reset, you have to control that door.

    - **The Drill:** Pick one hour today to put your phone in another room or turn on "Do Not Disturb."

- **The Challenge:** Don't check it "just once." Use that hour to focus entirely on yourself or your family. You are proving that you, not your phone, are in charge of your attention.

3. **The Mirror Affirmation**

Self-trust starts with how you speak to yourself when things go wrong.

- **The Drill:** Look in the mirror tonight before bed. Even if you had a bad day, find one small promise you actually kept.

- **The Challenge:** Say out loud: "I kept my word on [X], and I am becoming someone I can trust." It might feel silly at first, but you are rewiring your brain to look for your wins instead of your failures.

The "Push-Back" Reality Check

Expect people to be surprised. Some might even get upset. That's okay. Their reaction is about them; your boundary is about you.

- **Remember:** You aren't being mean; you are being **honest.** A "No" today prevents a blow-up tomorrow.

THE HARD QUESTIONS:
Seeing Your New Worth

Answer these questions to see the change happening in your life. Don't look for perfection; look for the small signs that you are moving out of the "Pain" and into your new "Home."

1. **What did I get back by saying "No"?** Think of a time you said "No" recently. Did it give you an hour of rest? Did it save you from a stressful argument?

   - **The Reality:** Every "No" to a distraction is a "Yes" to your own peace. You are finally making room for what truly matters.

2. **How does my body feel today?** When you were people-pleasing, you felt sick, tense, and tired. How do you feel now that you are being more honest with people?

   - **The Reality:** Notice the difference. If you feel even a little bit lighter or less "panicked," that is proof that honesty is healing you. Your body is relieved that you are finally standing up for yourself.

3. **Who is still standing by me?** We often worry that everyone will leave if we start setting boundaries. Look at the people who are still in your life right now.

   - **The Reality:** The people who truly care about you will respect your "No." You aren't losing friends; you are filtering for quality. You are discovering who your real tribe is.

4. **Whose respect matters most to me right now?** Are you still worried about what the "Joneses" think, or are you starting to care more about what the person in the mirror thinks?

   - **The Reality:** You are moving away from the need for everyone to like you. You are starting to value your own integrity more than the noise of the crowd.

5. **What is one promise I kept to myself this week?** Did you take that walk? Did you turn off your phone when you said you would?

   - **The Reality:** Celebrate that win. Keeping a promise to yourself is the fastest way to build **unshakable worth.** It proves you are someone you can finally trust.

The Reality of Your Growth

If you can see even a small change in these areas, you are no longer living in your old "home" of pain. You have moved out of the burnout and into a life where you are in control.

The weight is lifting because you stopped carrying everyone else's drama. You are walking a new path now, and every "No" is a step toward the person you were always meant to be.

THE COMMMITMENT:
My Promise to Me

For a long time, you have been the person everyone else could count on. You kept your promises to your boss, your friends, your family, your church and your neighbors, even when it made you tired or sick. Now, it is time to make a promise to the most important person in your life: **The person in the mirror.**

This isn't about being mean or selfish. It's about being healthy. When you are at peace, you are better for your family and for the world.

From now on, I make this commitment to myself:

- **I will be honest.** *I won't say "Yes" just to keep things quiet if I really mean "No." I would rather have a moment of awkwardness than a week of stress.*

- **I will protect my peace.** *I am the only one who can guard my time and energy. I will stop letting people use me like a doormat.*

- **I will start small.** *I will keep the little promises I make to myself. I know that every small win helps me trust myself again.*

- **I will stop comparing.** *I don't need to keep up with anyone else. I am focused on my own health and my own family and that is ok.*

The Step Forward

Take a breath and look in the mirror. Say this to yourself: **"I am done living for everyone else's rules. I am in charge of my own peace."**

Signed, ____________________________________

(*No more excuses. No more waiting. This is who I am now.*)

THE FINAL CHARGE:

Take Back Your Life

The time for talk is over. You have the roadmap, you have the tools, and you have the truth. Now, it is time to walk out the door and live it.

Don't wait for a "perfect time" to start saying no. Don't wait until you feel "ready" or "brave enough." Bravery doesn't come before the action, it comes because of the action. You will feel brave the moment you stand your ground for the first time.

Remember this as you go:

- **You are not "mean" for having limits.**
  You are human.

- **You are not "selfish" for needing peace.**
  You are wise.

- **You are not "failing" anyone by being honest.**
  You are finally being real.

The old home of pain, sickness, and people-pleasing is behind you. Every time you choose your peace over someone else's drama, you are walking further away from that old life. You are moving toward a life of **unshakable worth,** where your "Yes" means something because your "No" is firm.

Go out today and protect your peace. Keep that one small promise to yourself. Look the world in the eye and know that you are no longer a doormat, you are a person of strength.

The person in the mirror is finally looking back at you with a smile. Don't let them down.

THE SEAL:
A Prayer for Strength and Peace

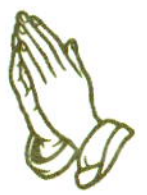

Dear Heavenly Father,

Thank You for the gift of peace and the strength to protect it. I confess that I have spent too much time trying to please others while neglecting the life You gave me. I have lived in the pain of "yes" for too long, and today I choose to move out of that old home.

Please give me the courage to be honest. When I am tempted to say "yes" out of fear or guilt, help me to pause and choose the truth instead. Strengthen my heart so that I can be a person of my word, to others and to myself. Help me to remember that my worth is found in You, not in how much I do for everyone else.

I commit my schedule, my family, and my peace to Your hands. Help me to walk forward with confidence, knowing that You are with me as I build this new life of unshakable worth.

In Jesus' name,
Amen

*"All you need to say is a simple 'Yes' or 'No';
anything beyond this comes from the evil one."*

— Matthew 5:37 NIV

My Notes

Date: ___________________

My Notes

Date: ___________________

My Notes

Date: ______________

My Notes

Date: ______________

PART THREE

Rebuild

Rising Above:
Walking Your Divine Assignment

CHAPTER 7

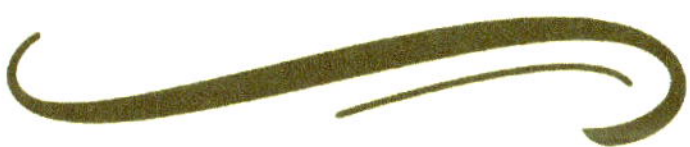

MOVE YOUR FEET

Purpose is found in motion, not in waiting.

THE INVITATION:
Leave the Waiting Room

You are cordially invited to stop waiting.

For too long, you have been waiting for permission to be happy. You've been waiting for someone to tell you that you've "healed enough" or that it's finally "your turn." You've been sitting in the waiting room of your own life, watching everyone else move forward while you managed the pain.

This is your official notice: The waiting room is closed.

I am inviting you to step into the unknown. It will feel a little uncomfortable, and that's okay. Comfort is what kept you stuck in your old habits. Growth lives in the movement.

You don't need to have a grand plan. You don't need to have a degree in "how to be perfect." You just need to accept this invitation to show up for yourself.

Will you accept? Will you agree that your life is worth more than just "getting by"? Will you decide right now that the person you are becoming is worth the risk of a first step?

Purpose is calling your name, but it won't come into the waiting room to find you. You have to meet it out on the path.

MY STORY:
The Confession:
The High Horse and the Waiting Room

For years, I told myself I was just "waiting for the right moment." I told myself I was waiting for the right person, the right job, or the right opportunity. But if I'm being honest with you, the kind of honesty that hurts, I was actually just expecting my life to drop out of the sky.

I used to pray and treat God like a spiritual ATM. I'd ask Him for everything I wanted without ever getting off my butt to put in the work. Does that shock you? Maybe. But how many of us have done the exact same thing? We pray for change, but we aren't willing to move a muscle to help ourselves.

I lived in a cycle of **entitlement.** I felt like I deserved the best, yet I did nothing to reach my goals. Instead, I spent my time:

- **Scrolling in Resentment:** I'd watch successful people on social media and feel a deep envy.

- **Throwing Pity Parties:** I'd slip into my corner, complaining and even gossiping about others just to make myself feel better.

- **Wearing the Mask:** Remember, I was the Queen of Masks. I didn't show this bitterness to the world; I was too busy "keeping up with the Joneses."

Inside, I was screaming: "When is it my turn? Why can't I be happy?"

I had to let go of my pride. I had to stop acting like a spoiled child and **repent.** It was confronting to realize that I had tried to fill the gaps in my soul with everything that was bad for me, a path that eventually led me to the edge of suicide.

Real change didn't happen until I broke down my pride and got professional help. With time, healing, the right mentors, and a real relationship with Jesus, I finally moved out of that "waiting room" of laziness, entitlement, and the blame game.

I started gaining new skills. I started building healthy habits. I stopped looking at what others had and started looking at what I could do. And guess what? When my focus shifted to what was good, the opportunities started to flow.

It wasn't easy. I was still fighting that "failure stack" I told you about. But step by step, with intentional choices, I walked out of the waiting room and into my purpose.

Here is the promise: When you commit your ways to the Lord, He will guide your steps. I am living proof of it, and He will do the exact same for you.

THE TRUTH:
You Are Not a Victim of Your Waiting

Here is the hard, beautiful truth: **The only person who can keep you in the waiting room is you.**

You've made it through the chapters on pain. You've learned how to say "No" and set boundaries. You've started to trust the person in the mirror. But now, we have to deal with the last hurdle, the belief that you aren't ready to be great.

We often stay stuck in our "home of pain" because it feels safe. We know how to be sad. We know how to be tired. We know how to complain. But moving into purpose? That requires us to put down the remote, stop the scrolling, and actually show up.

The Truth is this: God didn't save you from your past just so you could sit on the sidelines. He didn't pull you out of the pit just for you to find a "nicer" spot to sit still. He pulled you out so you could run your race. Your story of pain was never meant to be a life sentence; it was meant to be your **fuel.** All those years you spent being a doormat, all those nights you felt suicidal, and all those moments you felt "less than", those weren't for nothing. They were the lessons that gave you the strength to lead others.

Here is the shift you need to feel in your heart today:

- **You don't need** more "perfect circumstances."

- **You don't need** the approval of the people who used to walk all over you.

- **You don't need** to see the finish line to start the race.

You have a purpose that nobody else on this planet can fulfill. It isn't a generic plan; it was uniquely created just for you. You weren't born by accident, and you didn't survive your pain by sheer luck. You were created for this exact time and this very moment by a loving God who has been intentional about you from the start.

But here is the most important part:
Your movement isn't just about you anymore.

There is someone out there right now who is trapped in the same "waiting room" you just left. They are stuck in the same pain, the same people-pleasing, and the same hopelessness that used to be your home. They are waiting for someone to show them the way out, and that someone is **you.**

Your story is the map they need. Your scars are the proof they've been looking for that healing is possible. But you can't lead them to freedom if you are still sitting down. You can't help them find their way if you are still waiting for "permission" to move. When you move your feet, you aren't just walking toward your own future, you are clearing a path for the person behind you.

Purpose is not a destination you reach; it is a way you walk.

The change is happening. You can feel it. That "hissy fit" of resentment is being replaced by a hunger for growth. The envy of others is being replaced by the excitement for your own path. You are no longer a spoiled child waiting for a handout; you are a child of God stepping into an inheritance.

THE REALITY CHECK:
Motion vs. Meaningless Busywork

It is time for a real conversation. We often mistake "being busy" for "moving forward." You can spend all day scrolling through motivational quotes, bought-out journals, podcasts and "planning" your big life, but if your feet haven't moved, you are still in the waiting room.

Let's check the reality of where you are standing right now:

- **The Prayer Check:** Are you asking God to open doors while you are refusing to walk down the hallway? Prayer is a powerful steering wheel, but it doesn't do much if the engine isn't running.

- **The Social Media Check:** Are you using other people's success as an excuse to feel bad about yourself? If looking at someone else's life makes you bitter instead of inspired, it's time to put the phone down. You are wasting the energy you need for your own race by watching theirs.

- **The "Ready" Check:** Are you waiting for the fear to go away before you start? Reality check: **The fear doesn't leave until the action starts.** You don't get brave sitting on the couch; you get brave in the middle of the move.

- **The Entitlement Check:** Do you still feel like the world "owes" you something because you suffered? Pain is a terrible currency. You can't trade your past hurts for a future success. You have to build that future with the tools you have today.

The Bottom Line: You are no longer a victim of your past. **You are the architect of your today.** If you want a life of purpose, you have to stop waiting for a handout and start putting your hands to work.

The "Joneses" aren't your problem. Your "High Horse" isn't your problem. The only thing standing between you and your divine purpose is the decision to move your feet.

A Hard Truth to Swallow

If you stay where you are, you aren't just hurting yourself, you are leaving that person in the "waiting room" behind you without a guide. Your laziness or your fear is standing in the way of someone else's hope.

Is your comfort worth someone else's continued pain? I didn't think so. It's time to get up.

THE DRILL:
Time to Work

Thinking about your purpose is one thing, but practicing it is another. We are done with "someday." We are starting today. This drill is designed to push you out of the waiting room and get your feet on the path.

1. **The "Do It Anyway" Step**

    Pick one thing you've been avoiding because you're "scared" or "not ready." Maybe it's signing up for a class, making a difficult phone call, or finally starting that project or applying for a job. **Do it today.** Don't wait for the fear to go away, do it while you're shaking. That is how bravery is born.

2. **The Comparison Kill-Switch**

    For the next two days, **stay off social media entirely** unless it's for work. No scrolling, no checking, no "just one peek." Use that extra time to focus on *your* habits and *your* growth. You'll be amazed at how fast you can move when you stop looking at how fast everyone else is going.

3. **The Skill-Up Challenge**

What is one thing you need to learn to get to where you want to go? Spend 30 minutes today actually learning it. Read an article, watch a tutorial, or practice the craft. Stop talking about "gaining a skillset" and actually start building one.

4. **The "Hands-on" Service**

Find someone to help today, but do it from a place of strength, not people-pleasing. Offer a hand to someone who is struggling, not because you need them to like you, but because you are a person of value who has something to give. Movement is most powerful when it's used to lift others up.

THE HARD QUESTIONS:
Move Your Feet

1. **Are you hiding behind "God's timing" to avoid your own responsibility?**

    We love to say we are "waiting on the Lord" when, in reality, God is waiting on us to get out of the boat. If you've already been given the vision, why are you still asking for a sign?

    - **The Challenge:** Is your stillness actually faith, or is it just fear with a religious mask on it?

2. **If you died today, would your purpose die with you?**

    Purpose isn't something you *have*; it's something you *release* into the world. If you keep "planning" to be great but never move, the world misses out on what you were built to provide.

    - The Challenge: Are you okay with leaving your potential in the graveyard because you were too comfortable to start?

3. **Whose life is currently on hold because you refuse to get moving?**

There is someone out there who needs the solution you carry. They are waiting for the business you haven't started, the testimony you haven't shared, or the help you haven't offered. Your "waiting room" is their prison.

- **The Challenge:** Who is suffering right now because you're still "preparing" for a day that never comes?

4. **What is the one lie you tell yourself most often to justify staying still?**

"I don't have the money." "I'm not as good as them." "I'm waiting for the right season." We all have a favorite lie that helps us sleep at night while our dreams stay dusty.

- **The Challenge:** If that lie was taken away from you right now, what would your excuse be then?

5. **Do you actually want the purpose, or do you just want the applause?**

   Stop dreaming about the "big life" if you aren't willing to embrace the big grind. Everyone wants the influence and the victory lap, but almost nobody wants the sore feet, the lonely hours, and the quiet discipline it takes to get there. If you aren't willing to do the grueling work in the dark when no one is watching, you're just a fan of success, not a builder of it.

   - **The Challenge:** Are you brave enough to be a "nobody" who works while everyone else is sleeping, or are you too addicted to being noticed to actually be productive?

The Hard Truth: You don't need more "motivation." You need more movement. The floor is open, the hallway is clear, and the door is unlocked. The only thing missing is the sound of your footsteps.

THE COMMMITMENT:
No More Waiting Rooms

From this moment on, I agree to these terms:

- **I will stop waiting for "perfect."** *I will start moving even if I'm shaking, even if I'm tired, and even if I don't have all the answers yet.*

- **I will stop blaming my past.** *My history is a lesson, not a life sentence. I will stop using what happened to me as an excuse for what I'm not doing today.*

- **I will choose work over attention.** *I am willing to be a "nobody" who gets the job done rather than a "somebody" who just talks about it.*

- **I will remember who needs me.** *I recognize that my laziness or fear is holding someone else back. I am getting up so I can pull someone else up behind me.*

The Final Word

Purpose isn't a feeling I'm waiting for; it's a choice I'm making. I am done watching from the sidelines. Today, I move my feet.

One Last Thing

Don't just sign this and close the book. If you sign this and go back to scrolling on your phone, you are lying to yourself. Look at your signature. Now go do the first thing on your list. **Move.**

Signed, ______________________________________

(No more excuses. No more waiting. This is who I am now.)

THE FINAL CHARGE:
The Line in the Sand

There is no "Plan B." There is no going back to the person who sat around wondering "what if." or "the would have, could have, should have." You are now a person of movement.

Stop Asking for Permission

The world isn't going to hand you a trophy just for showing up. It's not going to ask you if you're ready. You have to take your place. Stop looking around for someone to tell you it's okay to start. Your purpose is your permission.

Stop Respecting Your Fear

Fear is a liar, but it's also a compass. Usually, the thing you are most afraid of is exactly what you need to do next. Don't wait for the fear to shrink; make your courage grow by moving right through the middle of it.

The Clock is Ticking

Every minute you spend "getting ready to get ready" is a minute you've stolen from the people you were meant to serve. Your purpose has an expiration date. Don't let yours die inside of you because you were too worried about being "prepared."

The Bottom Line

You aren't a victim of your circumstances. You aren't a slave to your past. And you aren't a spectator in this life. You are the driver.

The hallway is long, the work is hard, but the destination is divine. Stop talking. Stop planning. Stop waiting. It's time to move your feet.

THE SEAL:
A Prayer for the Path

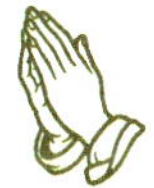

The Prayer

Heavenly Father,

I am tired of standing still. I have spent too much time in the waiting room, letting fear and "what-ifs" keep me from the life You designed for me. Today, I am putting my hands to work and my feet on the pavement.

Lord, I ask for the courage to be a "nobody" while I build what You've called me to build. When I am tempted to look at what others are doing, pull my eyes back to my own lane. When I feel like I don't have enough, remind me that You are the provider of the seed and the harvest.

I don't want to be "busy"; I want to be purposeful. I don't want to be "ready"; I want to be obedient. As I take these first messy, shaking steps, I trust that You are the one directing my path. Use my movement to bring hope to someone else and glory to Your name.

No more excuses. No more delays. I am moving now.

In Jesus Name, Amen.

*"Commit to the Lord whatever you do,
and He will establish your plans."*

— *Proverbs 16:3* NIV

My Notes

Date: ______________

My Notes

Date: _______________

My Notes

Date: ___________

My Notes

Date: _______________

CHAPTER 8

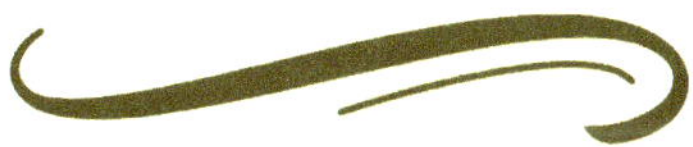

THE KEYS TO THE HOUSE

You don't live there anymore.

THE KEYS ARE YOURS
You are no longer a tenant in your pain

This is the final chapter, but it isn't the "end." It's your graduation. For this final section, we're changing the pace. I'm pulling up a chair right next to you. I'm not standing on a stage, and I'm not shouting from the finish line. I'm right here, shoulder to shoulder with you, looking at the road we've traveled.

We've done the hard work of **Releasing** the heavy weights, **Reclaiming** who you actually are, and **Rebuilding** a life that doesn't crumble.

Here is how we close this house and open your future.

A Letter to the Person You Used to Be

Before we take another step, I want you to take a second and look back at the version of you who first picked up this book.

Maybe that person was crying. Maybe they were numb. Maybe they felt like they were nothing more than the sum of their mistakes and their heartaches. I know that person well because I was that person, too.

I want you to tell that version of yourself: **"Thank you for not giving up on us."**

You see, for a long time, you lived in a house called "Pain." It was dark, the air was heavy, and you thought you had to stay there because you didn't think you deserved anything better. But look at your hands. You aren't holding onto those old walls anymore. You've walked out the front door.

The "Aha" Moment: You didn't read this book to find your worth. You read this book to realize that your worth was the ground you were standing on the whole time. You didn't "earn" it. You just finally cleared away the rubble so you could see it.

The Three Pillars of Your New Life

(How we live out *Release, Reclaim, and Rebuild* every single day)

1. The Daily Release (The Garden)

You are going to have bad days. People will still be unkind, and life will still be messy. But now, you have a "garden."

- **The Heart:** Instead of letting new pain into your house to rot, you put it in the garden. You use it as compost. You say, "This hurts, but it's just fuel for my growth." You don't let it sleep in your bed anymore.

2. The Daily Reclaim (The Foundation)

Every morning, you have to decide who defines you.

- **The Heart:** Your worth is "Unshakable." It's not based on your bank account, your relationship status, or how "productive" you were today. Your foundation is that you are a child of God, built with purpose. That doesn't change when the weather changes.

3. The Daily Rebuild (The Open Door)

Your new life isn't just for you to hide in. A beautiful home is meant for hosting.

- **The Heart:** Your "Divine Assignment" is simply this: Be a person who knows the way out. When you see someone else stuck in a "waiting room" or trapped in a house of pain, you don't judge them. You just show them your keys. You help them see that they can leave, too.

The Truth You Tell Yourself Every Morning

(Say this out loud every morning. For the men, let it be your shield. For the women, let it be your strength.)

- **I am not a guest in my own life; I am the owner.**

- **My past is a story I tell, not a place I live.**

- **I am not "recovering" from pain; I am living in my purpose.**

- **I have nothing to prove and everything to give.**

The Final Instruction: Your Turn to Write

You'll notice this chapter doesn't have as many pages as the others. That's because the rest of this story doesn't belong in this book. It belongs to you.

I've walked with you as far as I can. I've shared my heart, my scars, and the roadmap that saved my life. But now, the pen is in your hand.

The house is ready. The keys are yours. The door is open.

Rise and walk.

From My Heart to Yours, A Final Blessing as You Go

Before you close this cover and set this book on your shelf, I want to leave you with one final blessing.

May you never again mistake your **scars** for your **identity.** Those marks are not evidence of your shame; they are proof of your survival and the blueprints of your strength.

May you have the courage to walk through every door that God opens for you, even if your knees are shaking. May you remember that you are never walking alone, and you are never walking without a purpose.

When the world tries to tell you that you are "too much" or "not enough," may the truth of your **Unshakable Worth** rise up like a shield. May you find rest in the fact that your value was settled before you ever took a breath, and nothing you do, or that was done to you, can ever take it away.

May your hands be quick to help others, your heart be slow to judge, and your feet be ready to move.

You have **Released** the weight. You have **Reclaimed** the truth. You have **Rebuilt** the ruins.

I am so proud of how far you've come.

Now, go and live in the home you were always meant to inhabit.

Peace be with you on the journey.

You are loved. You are chosen. And you are finally home.

Pain Is No Longer Your Permanent Home. Freedom Is.

My Notes

Date: _______________

My Notes

Date: ___________

My Notes

Date: ______________

My Notes

Date: _______________

PART FOUR

Your Next Steps

Continuing the Journey

WALKING FORWARD

My friend, if you're looking for deeper guidance or community as you continue this journey, I'd love to walk alongside you.

1. The Commitment to Continued Growth

Healing isn't a destination; it's a commitment. As you move forward, keep these practices at the heart of your life:

- **Keep Writing Your Story:** The pages of this book may end, but your story doesn't. Keep journaling, reflecting, and setting new goals. Every step forward, no matter how small, is still progress.

- **Keep Walking with God:** You don't need fancy words. Just keep talking to Him honestly from your heart, He is waiting to hear from you. ***"Draw near to God, and He will draw near to you."*** — *James 4:8 NIV*

- **Surround Yourself with Support:** Healing thrives in safe spaces. Find a local church, a faith-based group, or people who uplift you and speak life into your journey. You were never meant to do this alone.

- **Take Care of Your Heart and Mind:** Be kind to yourself. Rest when you need to. Seek professional or pastoral help if you feel overwhelmed. Find a mentor, a coach or a friend you can trust. Your mental, emotional, and spiritual health all matter equally.

2. Walk It Out With Aroha: Coaching and Community

You've done the heart work, and I am so proud of you. If you are ready to convert these truths into sustained action, I invite you to explore deeper guidance:

- **Deeper Guidance:** You can join me in one of my coaching programs, 1:1 sessions, or workshops designed to help you rise stronger and live with purpose.

- **Stay Connected:** I'd love to keep walking with you as you grow in confidence, faith, and purpose. Stay connected for encouragement, new resources, and empowering programs.

To learn more and take your next step, please visit:

aroharipley.com

Follow: ***aroharipley*** on all social media platforms

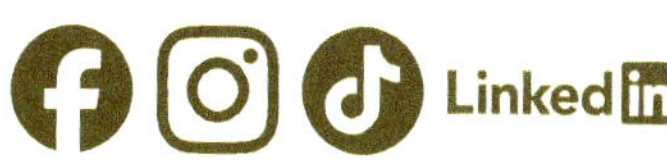

About the Author: Aroha Ripley

Aroha Ripley is not built on titles or polished narratives. She is a proud Indigenous Māori woman shaped by faith, whānau, and lived experience.

Before the coaching, the speaking, or the book, she is a wife, a mother, a nanny, a sister, and an aunty. Family is not something she fits in around her work, it is the foundation of how she lives. Legacy matters. Responsibility matters. People matter more than platforms.

Her life has been forged through pain, fear, and adversity, the kind that isn't visible but leaves its mark. She knows what it means to function while carrying unresolved pain, to survive seasons that demand strength before healing is available. Rather than allowing those experiences to harden her or define her, she faced them. That decision changed the trajectory of her life and the work she now does.

Aroha is a business and transformation coach, mentor, speaker, and author who works with both individuals and businesses. She refuses to soften the truth for comfort and believes real change begins with honesty, honesty about pain, patterns, and personal responsibility. Her work is faith-led, tested through experience, and informed by theory.

She is the author of *Sassy Lips, Fearless Queens*, a bold statement for women to stop shrinking and reclaim their voice, confidence, and purpose. Through her work, Aroha challenges people to confront what they've avoided, take ownership of their healing, and live in alignment with who they were created to be.

Aroha's story is not one of perfection or arrival. It is one of choosing to rise, again and again, with integrity, courage, and truth, even when it costs comfort.

To find out more visit the websites:

artalentmanagementagency.com
and
aroharipley.com

A NOTE OF FAITH: Prayer Invitation

Maybe you don't know Jesus, or you're not sure if He could love you after all you've been through. But let me tell you, He already does. He's been with you in the hardest moments, and He's never left your side.

If you've never invited Jesus into your life, this could be the moment everything changes. It's not about fancy words; it's about an open heart, a relationship with Him.

You can pray this right now:

A Prayer Invitation

Prayer of Invitation: Come As You Are

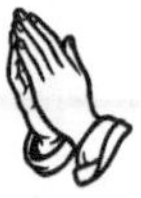

Dear Jesus,

I'm tired of trying to do life on my own. I've searched for peace in so many places, but nothing has filled the emptiness inside me. Today, I open my heart to You. I may not have all the words, but I know I need You. I believe You are real, that You love me just as I am, and that You gave Your life so I could be free. Please forgive me for my sins and wash away the pain and mistakes I've carried. I choose to let go of what's behind me and welcome the new life You have for me. Come into my heart, Jesus. Be my Lord, my peace, and my strength. Teach me how to walk with You each day. Thank You for giving me a fresh start.

In Jesus' Name,

Amen

If you prayed this for the first time, know this: **you are now God's child, deeply loved, fully forgiven, and never alone.** If you took this step today, I would love to welcome you and celebrate with you.

Aroha xx

CRISIS SUPPORT NUMBERS

CRISIS HELPLINES

If you are in immediate danger, please contact your local emergency services immediately. Reaching out is not weakness—it's courage. It may be the first step toward the healing and freedom you truly deserve.

Australia

- Lifeline: **13 11 14**
  24/7 crisis support and suicide prevention

- Beyond Blue: **1300 22 4636**
  mental health support

- 1800 RESPECT: **1800 737 732**
  24/7 family, domestic & sexual violence support

New Zealand

- Lifeline NZ: **0800 543 354** or free text **4357 (HELP)**

- Need to Talk?: Free call or text **1737**
  24/7 with a trained counsellor

- Women's Refuge: **0800 733 843**
  support for women experiencing family violence

United States

- 988 Suicide & Crisis Lifeline: Dial **988**
  24/7 crisis support

- National Domestic Violence Hotline:
  1-800-799-7233 or text "START" to **88788**

United Kingdom

- Samaritans: **116 123**
  24/7 for anyone in emotional distress

- National Domestic Abuse Helpline:
  0808 2000 247
  24/7 support for women experiencing abuse

Please note: Numbers may change over time. If you're unsure, please search for the most up-to-date crisis support services in your country.